the
CULTURED COOK

the
CULTURED COOK

DELICIOUS FERMENTED FOODS

with Probiotics to Knock Out Inflammation, Boost Gut Health, Lose Weight & Extend Your Life

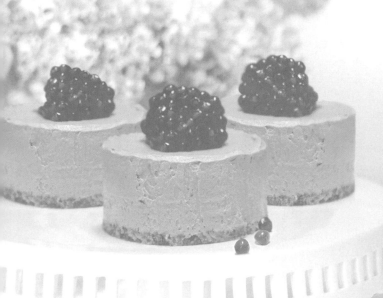

MICHELLE SCHOFFRO COOK, PhD, DNM

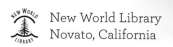 New World Library
Novato, California

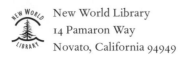 New World Library
14 Pamaron Way
Novato, California 94949

The material in this book is intended for education. No expressed or implied guarantee of the effects of the use of the recommendations can be given or liability taken. It is not meant to take the place of diagnosis and treatment by a qualified medical practitioner or therapist.

Text design by Tona Pearce Myers and Megan Colman
Recipe photographs by Michelle Schoffro Cook

Library of Congress Cataloging-in-Publication Data
Names: Cook, Michelle Schoffro, author.
Title: The cultured cook : delicious fermented foods with probiotics to knock out inflammation, boost gut health, lose weight, and extend your life / Michelle Schoffro Cook, PhD, DNM.
Description: Novato, California : New World Library, 2017. | Includes bibliographical references and index.
Identifiers: LCCN 2017018859 (print) | LCCN 2017027740 (ebook) | ISBN 9781608684861 (Ebook) | ISBN 9781608684854 (alk. paper)
Subjects: LCSH: Probiotics. | Fermented foods—Health aspects. | Fermented foods—Recipes.
Classification: LCC RM666.P835 (ebook) | LCC RM666.P835 C65 2017 (print) | DDC 641.3/7—dc23
LC record available at https://lccn.loc.gov/2017018859

First printing, September 2017
ISBN 978-1-60868-485-4
Ebook ISBN 978-1-60868-486-1
Printed in Canada

 New World Library is proud to be a Gold Certified Environmentally Responsible Publisher. Publisher certification awarded by Green Press Initiative. www.greenpressinitiative.org

10   9   8   7   6   5   4   3   2   1

*I dedicate this book to
my wonderful and loving husband, Curtis
(whatever souls are made of, yours and mine are the same),
and my supportive and loving parents, Michael and Deborah Schoffro.*

CONTENTS

Chapter 7. Recipes for Using Your Cultured Creations 155

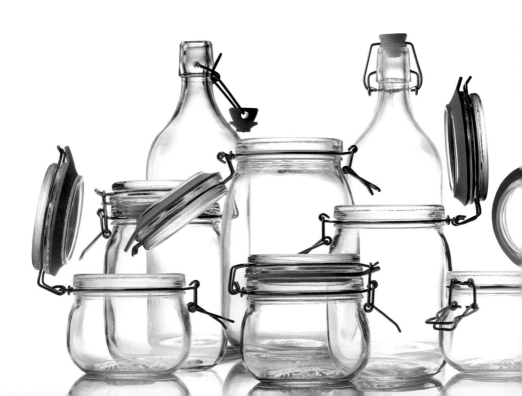

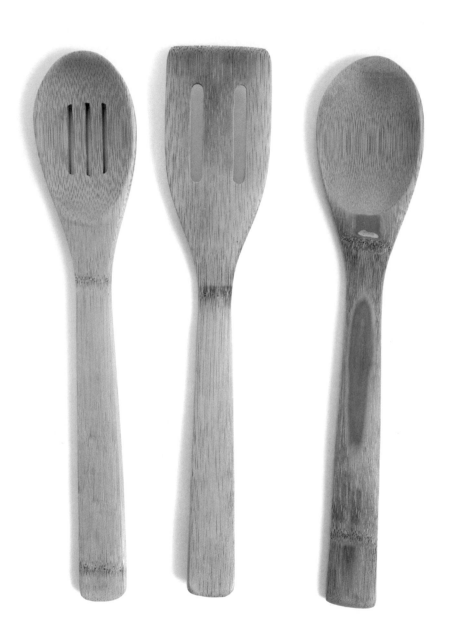

CHAPTER ONE

FERMENTED FOODS

The Missing Ingredient to Amazing Health

I am passionate about fermented foods. I love making them, eating them, and inventing new ones. My kitchen routinely bustles with microbial activity and new cultured creations. I've even reserved one counter as a fermentation station. Almost daily we eat at least one kind of fermented food, from sauerkraut to cheesecake and ice cream (yes, cheesecake *and* ice cream, which are among my favorite fermented food innovations!). Just ask my husband, Curtis, who enjoys my sauerkraut so much I've nicknamed him Krautis. He often comments that we share our kitchen (and sometimes our living room and dining room too, if I can't find kitchen space for my crocks!) with millions of microbes working their magic. He doesn't mind, though, because he knows that our little microbe community results in a wide variety of delicious and health-building food that we both enjoy.

Our friend Craig Sibley, co-owner of A-bun-dance Artisanal Bakery and Café in Lillooet, BC, Canada, with his wife, Dana, told me that it was clear from my kitchen — and the many ferments under way — that I am a mad scientist. Dana excitedly runs to the fermented foods workstation in my kitchen every time she visits to check out the various cultured creations in progress. She tells me that I am an alchemist, transforming everyday foods into even more nutritious and delicious ones.

Now I would like to share my handiwork to show *you* how you can take everyday foods and transform them into delicious superfoods at home in your kitchen with minimal effort and almost no money! It's true! Simply by fermenting vegetables, nuts, beans, and other foods into sauerkraut, yogurt, kimchi, and more, you significantly multiply their health-building properties.

It is my goal not only to teach you about some of the amazing health benefits of common fermented foods, but also to show you how easy it is to make them at home. Additionally, I will show you how you can take your fermented food creations to the next level, elevating them to include fermented foods you've probably never heard of before: probiotic-rich dairy-free cheeses, fermented cheesecakes, cultured ice cream, cultured fruit chutneys, and fermented salsas, to name a few. You'll soon learn that everyday foods like yogurt and sauerkraut are just the beginning of what is possible. You'll discover how easy it is to make fermented foods that boost the flavor of your meals, and you might even find some new favorite foods too.

No matter how delicious these cultured creations may taste, the reality is that there is far more to eating fermented foods than their great taste — there are also some incredible health benefits. And while most people are familiar with the gut-boosting properties of these cultured creations, their healing properties go well beyond the gut. Some of these health benefits include cancer prevention and healing, diabetes reduction, and a boost in immunity against many other diseases. Research shows that some fermented foods like kimchi and sauerkraut may even help in the fight against superbugs — those virulent strains of bacteria, viruses, and fungi that have become stronger and are now resistant to most of our medicines — when our best antibiotics fail!

I'm certainly not claiming that fermented foods are cures for whatever ails you, but I would be remiss if I didn't include some of the exciting research that shows the tremendous potential of fermented foods and the many probiotics they contain. Although probiotics are often touted as "beneficial bacteria," that is technically an incomplete description. It is true that many beneficial bacteria are considered probiotics, but that is only part of the story: probiotics can also include other types of beneficial microbes like yeasts. Probiotics are any of the vast number and variety of living microorganisms that bestow health benefits when ingested in food (or taken in supplement form, if you choose to do so).

When I mention beneficial yeasts, people immediately assume that all yeasts cause yeast infections. But they don't — probiotic yeasts do not cause infections. Actually, more and more research shows that probiotic yeasts may help your body address harmful yeast infections.

I also frequently hear people who consider themselves "in the know" tell me, "I get all the probiotics I need from eating yogurt every day," or something to that effect. They claim they don't need any other fermented foods in their diet. Although a good-quality yogurt that contains live cultures certainly confers some health benefits, in reality yogurt is not enough on its own because it typically contains only a few of strains of probiotics, and some types of commercially available yogurt don't contain any live cultures at all.

Even if you eat a high-quality yogurt with live cultures every day, you will benefit from getting a wider variety of probiotic strains in your diet. Our bodies naturally need many different strains of probiotics to help us maintain our health. Getting a couple of strains from yogurt is a good first step to restoring the beneficial microbes in the body, but it is just a first step. Eating a wide variety of probiotics from a range of fermented foods can assist you on your quest for great health.

It really doesn't matter whether you're trying to prevent or fight diseases like diabetes and cancer or simply trying to maintain great health. Regardless of your health goals, fermented foods can likely help, at least to some degree. That's because a growing body of exciting research shows that these foods and the beneficial probiotics they contain boost your immune system, increase your energy, and even prevent and heal many diseases, including Alzheimer's disease and other brain diseases, anxiety, cancer, depression, and heart disease, to name just a few. It's no surprise that fermented foods are the hottest topic in the field of health right now.

In this chapter and throughout *The Cultured Cook* I'll explain the most common methods of fermenting foods, detail why fermented foods transform everyday foods into superfoods, and explore the many health benefits of eating fermented foods on a regular basis.

You'll learn everything you need to know to get started with fermenting delicious and nutritious foods in your home kitchen. I'll share step-by-step instructions on how to ferment your own foods, including sauerkraut, kimchi, salsa, chutney, kombucha (a natural fermented soda traditionally made from tea, but you can also use coffee), dairy-free yogurt, vegan kefir (a fermented beverage), and vegan cheeses. I'll share many of my favorite recipes, like World's Easiest Yogurt, Walnut Thyme Cheese, Chèvrew (my dairy-free take on chèvre), Macadamia Cream Cheese, African Red Tea Kombucha, Spiced Sauerkraut, White Kimchi, Salvadoran Salsa, Red-Hot Hot Sauce, Cultured Spicy Peach Chutney, Gingerbread Cookie Ice Cream Sandwiches, Pumpkin Pie Ice Cream, Orange Creamsicle Cheesecake, and Dairy-Free Pomegranate Cheesecake.

Regardless of your dietary needs, rest assured that all the recipes in this book are plant based and suitable for vegan diets. Additionally, they are all gluten-free and dairy-free, so if you have trouble with gluten or dairy, you'll still be able to enjoy the many recipes found here. Of course, if you eat wheat, meat, poultry, fish, or dairy products, you don't have to give up these foods as you start eating more fermented foods. Either way, you can still reap the health and culinary benefits of eating more plant-based, gluten-free, dairy-free fermented foods.

In addition to recipes for making your own fermented foods, I also share many recipes for *using* your fermented food creations, including Coconut Cream Cheese Frosting, Mixed Green Salad with Grilled Peaches and Chèvrew, Cardamom Pear Crêpes with Macadamia Cream Cheese, and many others. Actually, in chapter 8 you'll discover twenty-five ways to enjoy more fermented foods in your diet — ways that go beyond yogurt or sauerkraut on hot dogs.

In *The Cultured Cook* I am happy to share the exciting research into how fermented foods can help to heal your gut, which, you may be surprised to learn, is a factor for most people suffering from almost any chronic health condition. I will share how healing your gut can alleviate the inflammation in your whole body, which is a good thing too because inflammation is now considered a major factor in over one hundred health conditions. Eating more fermented foods will also help you lose weight without dieting (if you are overweight), protect you against superbugs (even when they are resistant to antibiotics), prevent cancer, and so much more.

I wanted to give you the tools you need to become more engaged on your healing path and to feel more empowered in your own kitchen by making and eating a wide variety of fermented foods. I created *The Cultured Cook* because I was disappointed in the lack of awareness about the myriad health benefits of fermented foods even though there is plenty of research on the subject in scientific journals; most books briefly described gut health, but that is only the tip of the iceberg when it comes to fermented foods. Additionally, I found minimal, if any, information in other fermented food books about making plant-based yogurts and cheeses packed with probiotics. Lastly, I also wanted to create recipes that elevated the flavors of fermented foods to new and exciting levels. Whenever I've shared my fermented food creations with friends they've been astounded to learn that these are plant-based foods that are healthy for them. And let's face it: I wanted a book that included ice cream — delicious, creamy, dairy-free, probiotic-rich ice cream. I knew it was a tall order, but I hope you'll be happy with the results.

Introducing Fermented Foods

Here is a brief introduction to some of the fermented foods you will discover in *The Cultured Cook*:

Yogurt. No fermented foods recipe book would be complete without instructions on how to make yogurt! In chapter 2, "Dairy-Free Yogurt," I'll be sharing the traditional method (though I've changed it to be dairy-free) as well as my own techniques that actually reduce the work and mess of yogurt making. You'll discover some of the many health benefits of regular yogurt consumption, including its ability to help reduce cholesterol and normalize blood sugar levels. Yogurt consumption has also been found to reduce homocysteine levels, and this in turn reduces the risk of health conditions like heart attack, stroke, and diabetes, all of which are linked to high levels of this compound. You'll even learn how regular yogurt consumption also helps to reduce the frequency and duration of respiratory infections. I'll share my recipes for Cultured Coconut Cream, Dairy-Free Cream, and more. But perhaps the most exciting thing I'll share in the chapter on yogurt is my fermentation discovery that makes light work of plant-based yogurt. Forget expensive yogurt-making machines or straining curds and whey like you need to do with dairy-based yogurt — my plant-based yogurt is faster, is easier, and involves less mess.

Cheese. While traditional cheeses have few, if any, probiotic benefits, I have developed unique vegan cheeses rich in health-boosting microbes that are so good, you won't miss the less-healthy dairy options. In chapter 3, "Vegan Cheeses," you'll find many delightful dairy-free cheeses that are easy to make, including Almond Farmer's Cheese, Walnut Thyme Cheese, Bracotta Cheese, Chèvrew, Aged Smoked Cheese, and more. Although other books offer vegan cheeses, sadly, most of these cheeses do not contain any probiotics at all — even if the authors added them in the recipes. That's because they are often heated or prepared in such a way as to destroy the probiotics they may have started with. As an alternative, I developed cheeses that ensure the viability of the beneficial bacteria, while I also made every effort to improve upon the flavors of vegan cheeses. I've had my share of rubbery vegan cheeses that simply do not please the palate, and I hope to help you avoid those nasty cheeses.

In chapter 4, "Sauerkraut, Pickles, and Cultured Vegetables," you'll discover how to make kimchi, naturally fermented pickles, sauerkraut, and other condiments.

Kimchi, the national dish of Korea, is typically a fermented mixture of cabbage, chilis, and garlic. There are more than two hundred classic varieties of kimchi found in Korea, but there are probably as many variations on the dish as there are Koreans who make it. Research at Georgia State University found that *L. plantarum*, the probiotic culture found in kimchi (as well as sauerkraut) confers protection against the flu and superbugs by regulating the body's innate immunity. In *The Cultured Cook* you'll enjoy my not-so-spicy White Kimchi recipe.

Pickles. Unfortunately, most pickles found in grocery stores have been pasteurized and therefore do not have any probiotics, if they ever had them at all. The process of pickling foods in white vinegar does not help to develop probiotic cultures; however, fermenting vegetables using certain probiotic-promoting processes develops beneficial bacteria and some yeasts that also boost health. Additionally, the process of commercially preparing foods for grocery store shelves involves killing all bacteria — good or bad — to extend their shelf life. Making your own is the best way to ensure you're getting lots of probiotics. Besides that, the unique and wide range of flavors of homemade, fermented pickles is unbeatable. You'll enjoy Spicy Dill Fermented Pickles, Zucchini Pickles, Red-Hot Hot Sauce, Taco Pickles, and other amazing cultured vegetables.

Sauerkraut is one of the most overlooked yet research-proven superfoods. The natural probiotics found in this German staple, including *Lactobacillus plantarum* and *L. mesenteroides*, actually help to fight off harmful *E. coli* infections. *L. plantarum* has antiviral effects, making it a potential ally in treating colds, the flu, Ebola, HIV, chronic fatigue syndrome, and other viral conditions. You'll savor Basic Sauerkraut, Spiced Sauerkraut, Five-Minute Broccoli Sauerkraut, and other delightful creations.

Curtido, a Salvadoran condiment, is essentially a cross between salsa and kimchi. Like kimchi, it is packed with a wide range of probiotic strains and has many immune-boosting, superbug-fighting, anticancer health benefits. Once you've tried my favorite fermented food, Salvadoran Salsa (enhanced with turmeric and green apple), you'll be adding it to every meal.

Fruit Cultures. In chapter 5, "Fruit Cultures and Homemade Vinegar," you'll learn how to make fermented chutneys and fruit toppings for ice cream, toast, or yogurt, as well as fruit vinegars. You'll enjoy such recipes as Cultured Spicy Peach Chutney, Sweet Vanilla Peaches, Crabapple Vinegar, and other fruit vinegars.

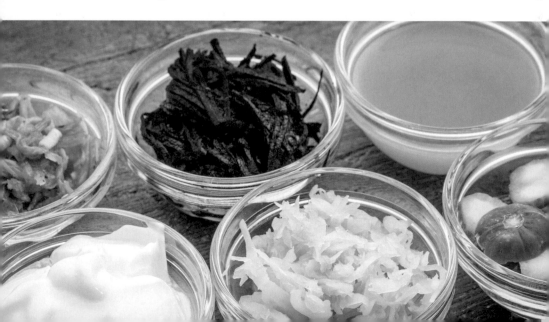

In chapter 6, "Cultured Beverages: Vegan Kefir, Kombucha, and More," you'll learn how to make cultured beverages, including kefir and kombucha. They make excellent fermented replacements for basic juices and unhealthy sodas. You'll also learn how to make my delicious Cultured Nonalcoholic Bloody Mary.

Kefir (pronounced *ke-FEER*) is similar to a drinkable form of yogurt but is so much healthier, thanks to having ten different probiotic strains compared to yogurt's one or two. It naturally contains B vitamins that give an energy boost, aid digestion, and help to regulate blood sugar and cholesterol levels. You'll love my Vegan Kefir and how it will make you feel.

Kombucha (pronounced *kom-BOO-shuh*) is an effervescent, natural soda-type beverage believed to have originated in Russia and China over two thousand years ago, although the exact origin is unknown. According to research, consuming kombucha could potentially prevent a broad spectrum of metabolic and infectious disorders while significantly improving digestion. Enjoy African Red Tea Kombucha as well as other natural sodas.

In chapter 7, "Recipes for Using Your Cultured Creations," you'll discover recipes that incorporate the wide variety of fermented foods you've learned how to make in the previous chapters. You'll also learn twenty-five ways to get more fermented foods into your daily diet. You'll love making recipes like Tzatziki (Greek-style yogurt cucumber dip), Cardamom Pear Crêpes with Macadamia Cream Cheese, Gingerbread Cookie Ice Cream Sandwiches, Orange Creamsicle Cheesecake, and Pumpkin Pie Ice Cream. I hope that the wide variety of treats I share will help you discover just how enjoyable eating fermented foods can be.

Why Maintaining a Healthy Gut Is the Key to Great Health — and How Fermented Foods Can Help

When was the last time you thought about your gut health? If you're like most people, you probably don't think much about it until you experience bloating, cramping, or indigestion. But more and more research is showing that great health begins in the gut. Here are some of the benefits of maintaining a healthy gut and enjoying more fermented foods.

Nutrient Absorption

Nutrients needed to build every cell in your body are absorbed through the walls of your gut. When you eat food, it is broken down into the foundational nutrients, which include amino acids (from protein), fatty acids (from fats), sugars (from carbohydrates), vitamins, minerals, enzymes (specialized proteins that aid digestion and other bodily functions), and phytonutrients (which literally means plant nutrients, such as lycopene in tomatoes or proanthocyanidins in blueberries, to cite only two of the thousands of phytonutrients in our food), among others. When these nutrients reach the gut they travel directly across the intestinal walls into the bloodstream, where they continue their journey to the brain, bones, heart, liver, or other parts that need replenishing. If the gut is compacted with waste products or the gut wall has become damaged, then no matter how many nutrients you obtain in your food or supplements, they won't make their way in sufficient amounts into your blood.

Preventing Inflammation

The gut determines whether we'll experience inflammation there or somewhere else in our bodies due to the permeability of the intestinal walls and the bacteria that reside there, which we'll discuss later in this chapter. If the gut wall becomes too permeable as a result of antibiotic use, excessive hormones, stress, poor diet, or other potential causes, whole food molecules — not just the nutrients — or waste matter can travel into the bloodstream. Because these food molecules and waste materials are not supposed to be in the blood, the immune system goes on alert and attacks them, causing low-grade, ongoing inflammation that can damage the body's cells and tissues, making them more vulnerable to illness.

Probiotic-Specific Benefits

The gut houses the bulk of the bacteria in our bodies — and we have more bacteria than cells in our bodies. The average person has approximately 100 trillion bacteria in her body, while she has about 50 to 100 trillion human cells. Although that may sound scary, these bacteria are largely beneficial or neutral in nature. Without these beneficial bacteria we could not live. These probiotics, as they are known, fight disease, ensure the digestion of food, manufacture nutrients, and kill nasty intruders that intend you harm. According to research in the medical journal *Internal and Emergency Medicine*, some of these bacteria help us to maintain a healthy weight.[1] Other research, published in the *Journal of Applied Microbiology*, shows that some probiotics kill harmful infections, even ones that reside in other parts of the body such as the lungs.[2] Still other probiotics in the gut have been shown in the *International Archives of Allergy and Immunology* to prevent or reduce allergic reactions.[3] And you can boost your gut health by increasing your consumption of probiotic-rich fermented foods.

Immune System Balancing

The gut is the site of a significant portion of the immune system, which helps keep us strong and healthy. By maintaining the gut, we may be able to boost our immune system to not only help prevent illness but also balance the way the immune system reacts to our own tissues and cells, and this in turn may beneficially affect autoimmune disorders. In autoimmune conditions the body attacks its own tissues as though they were foreign invaders like harmful pathogens; the type of autoimmune condition is determined by the type of tissue being attacked. Before you grab that decongestant to subdue your sinus congestion or antihistamine to stop the sneezing linked to spring allergies, you might want to give your gut some attention. More and more research shows that probiotic consumption can reduce allergy symptoms and, if started early in life, may even prevent allergic conditions altogether. But not just any probiotic will do: with thousands of probiotic strains available, it is important to choose the ones that have an anti-allergy effect. The right probiotic strains can not only heal the intestinal walls and reduce low-grade inflammation in the gut but also prevent, reduce, or delay allergy symptoms.[4]

Killing Superbugs

We've been engaging in a warfare of sorts against bacteria that are quickly learning to outsmart our weapons of choice: antibiotics. Consider that more than 70 percent of all bacterial infections in hospitals are resistant to at least one of the antibiotics used to treat them, according to the Food and Drug Administration (FDA).[5] But there is an interesting plot twist in this war: new players have emerged in the form of probiotics and the forgotten fermented foods of our ancestors. We more often consider probiotics for gut health and to prevent antibiotic-induced diarrhea, but a growing body of research now points to probiotics as potentially beneficial against superbugs. Research shows that some probiotics are helpful against resistant infections like *H. pylori* (linked to ulcers and other conditions) and MRSA (methicillin-resistant staphylococcus aureus), a serious and sometimes life-threatening infection primarily linked to hospital stays.[6] While antibiotics only attempt to kill the bacteria in one way, probiotics found in fermented foods have been found to fight MRSA infections in three ways: first, they compete with infectious bacteria for nutrients; second, they secrete bacteria-killing compounds known as bacteriocins; and third, they prevent infectious bacteria from producing a protective coating known as a biofilm. And bacterial infections are just the beginning: probiotics found in fermented foods are also showing potency against fungal infections — better known as yeast infections.[7]

Disease Prevention

Harmful infections in the gut can cause widespread inflammation. Consider rheumatoid arthritis, a body-wide autoimmune disorder in which the body attacks its own joints. Researchers at the New York University School of Medicine linked the disease to infectious intestinal bacteria known as *Prevotella copri*, speculating that the disease may begin in the gut, setting off an inflammatory response that spreads throughout the body.[8] Conversely, if the disease begins in the gut, its healing may also begin by healing the gut.

Brain Health Protection

The gut is increasingly becoming known as the "second brain" in medical circles as more and more research shows that gut health plays a significant role in brain health. Some probiotics found in the gut can function as antioxidants — nutrients that quell harmful free radicals before they can cause damage to the body's cells. These antioxidant probiotics may help protect the fatty parts of the brain from damage, and this in turn may help prevent brain diseases like Alzheimer's disease, Parkinson's disease, Lou Gehrig's disease, dementia, or others. The research into the effects of probiotics on brain health is still fairly early, but the promise and wide-reaching implications it holds is exciting. One preliminary animal study published in *BioMed Research International* found that certain naturally occurring probiotics in the gut can have a protective effect on cognitive function.[9] And according to research published in the medical journal *Nutrition Research*, the addition of more probiotics in the diet could help treat brain disorders like anxiety and depression.[10] Other research suggests that the brain benefits of ingesting more probiotics are sufficient to warrant including probiotics in the treatment plans of those suffering from Alzheimer's disease.[11] (To learn more about the benefits of fermented foods against anxiety, check out the sidebar below.)

Fermented Foods Alleviate Anxiety

If I told you that bacteria could alleviate your anxiety, you'd probably think I was joking or uninformed. But if you suffer from anxiety, particularly social anxiety, you'll be happy to learn about the exciting study conducted by researchers at the College of William and Mary in Williamsburg, Virginia. The study, published in *Psychiatry Research*, found that regularly consuming fermented foods replete with plentiful amounts of beneficial bacteria may indeed help reduce social anxiety.[12]

In the College of William and Mary study 710 students completed food diaries about their intake of fermented foods over the previous thirty days. They were also asked about exercise frequency and their consumption of fruits and vegetables so the researchers could control for healthy habits beyond fermented food intake. Researchers found that those who ate higher amounts of fermented foods had lower levels of social anxiety. The link was particularly noticeable among those who demonstrated signs of neuroticism.

Matthew Hilimire, a professor of psychology at the College of William and Mary and one of the researchers who conducted the study, said in an interview with *PsychCentral*, "It is likely that the probiotics in the fermented foods are favorably changing the environment in the gut, and changes in the gut in turn influence social anxiety."[13] The study found that people prone to anxiety experience less social anxiety when they frequently consume fermented foods replete with probiotics.

It may be hard to comprehend how bacteria can affect your mind, but an increasing body of research is proving that they do. A study conducted by researchers at McMaster University in Hamilton, Canada, published in the medical journal *Gastroenterology*, showed that the specific probiotic known as *Bifidobacterium longum* eliminated anxiety and normalized behavior. The researchers found that chronic gastrointestinal inflammation induces anxiety-like behavior and alters the biochemistry of the central nervous system.[14]

Further, a French study published in the *British Journal of Nutrition* confirms both the American and Canadian studies. They found that the same probiotic strain studied by the McMaster researchers, *B. longum*, along with another probiotic strain known as *Lactobacillus helveticus*, reduced anxiety. Additionally, the French study found that these two probiotics reduced psychological stress, depression, and feelings of anger and hostility.[15]

Although the exact mechanism or mechanisms at work are not yet clear, researchers believe that the probiotics reduce gastrointestinal inflammation and boost serotonin levels. Serotonin, a feel-good brain hormone sometimes called the happiness hormone, was once believed to be exclusively found in the brain but is actually produced by the gut; in fact, scientists estimate that about 90 percent of the body's serotonin can actually be found in the gastrointestinal (GI) tract. That's right: your intestines do some of the same work as your brain. And this is why many scientists now refer to the gut as the body's "second brain": the gut-brain health link has been the focus of a growing body of research proving the connection.

Weight Loss

Have you been trying to lose weight, counting calories, and exercising, but neither the scale nor pounds budge? A common problem of weight-loss programs that don't work or work for the short term but don't offer any lasting results is their failure to explore the link between gut health and weight loss. One of the keys to permanent weight loss is a healthy gut with plentiful amounts and a wide variety of strains of beneficial probiotics. Simply adding more fermented foods to your daily diet can make the difference.

In many studies the intestines of overweight and obese people were found to differ from those of lean people. Obese and overweight people tend to have a higher ratio of harmful microbes to beneficial ones.[16] The specific harmful microbes may differ from study to study, but the general consensus is that bad bugs (or a lack of good bacteria caused by insufficient amounts of fermented foods) may be making us fat. After all, most of our ancestors included fermented foods in their diet on a daily basis. Of course, overeating, poor eating choices, and inadequate physical activities are also responsible, but to adequately address weight issues it is important to eliminate from our bodies harmful pathogens that cause weight gain. And the best way to do that is to eat more fermented foods.

Many studies now show that the ratio of healthy bacteria to harmful microbes in our gut can influence our weight in several ways, including:

- Providing us with the energy we need through the breakdown of starches and sugars in our diet. Beneficial bacteria assist with digesting and absorbing these carbohydrates.
- Affecting cellular energy levels of liver and muscle cells. If the liver and muscles do not receive the energy they need to perform optimally, they don't function adequately and cannot break down fat stores and build up muscles that, in turn, break down fat.
- Affecting the accumulation of fat in our tissues.[17]

You're probably wondering if eating more fermented foods will really make much of a difference to your weight. Research shows that it does. A study published in the journal *Internal and Emergency Medicine* showed promising results in preventing and treating obesity and related metabolic disorders simply by changing the balance of intestinal flora in favor of the healthy probiotics found in many fermented foods.[18] In that study scientists examined the effects of administering probiotics to obese individuals. They found that probiotics could stabilize blood sugar levels; doing so reduces not only cravings for sweets and fatty foods but also the body's production of fat storage hormones. This combination results in a fat-melting alchemy that may help overweight and obese individuals lose weight even when other avenues aren't working. The study concluded that probiotics show promise in the prevention and treatment of obesity and metabolic disorders.[19]

But that's not all: insulin resistance is a common issue in overweight and obese individuals, a condition in which the body's cells aren't responding properly to the hormone insulin, which is secreted by the pancreas in response to sugars and starches in the diet. Unfortunately, insulin resistance increases the risk of metabolic syndrome, heart disease, type 2 diabetes, and obesity. Here's what happens: When you eat sweets or refined starches, blood sugar levels skyrocket. Because high blood sugar levels can be dangerous, especially to the brain, the pancreas — a long, thin organ just under the lower ribs on the left-hand side of the body — secretes insulin. The insulin then helps to lower blood sugar levels, but it also triggers fat storage in the body. Your blood sugar levels may then drop too low, causing cravings for sweets, bread, pastries, or other refined sugars and starches. You eventually give in to the cravings, causing a vicious cycle of excessive consumption of sweets and a blood-sugar roller coaster. Over time your cells lose their ability to respond to insulin and become resistant to it, and the body no longer transports sugar from the blood to the muscles or tissues where it is needed for energy, often resulting in metabolic syndrome.

Metabolic syndrome, also sometimes called syndrome X, is a collection of symptoms linked with insulin resistance. Metabolic syndrome is frequently linked to high blood pressure, low HDL cholesterol (known as the "good cholesterol"), and an increased risk of blood clotting. The World Health Organization characterizes metabolic syndrome as including all the following symptoms:

- high blood pressure (140/90 mmHg or above) or being treated for high blood pressure
- abdominal obesity, which is usually described as a waist measurement above 37 inches
- high insulin levels after fasting or after meals
- high triglyceride levels (at least 150 mg/dL) or HDL cholesterol levels lower than 35 mg/dL

Although health professionals recognize the importance of eating a healthy diet and exercising to restore the body to a healthier weight, few realize the importance of a healthy balance of beneficial bacteria to pathogenic ones in the treatment of insulin resistance, metabolic syndrome, overweight and obesity, and type 2 diabetes. Consider the effects on obese laboratory rats when scientists examined the effects of probiotics. Obese rats eating a high-fat diet were divided into a control group and a second group that was given two strains of beneficial bacteria on a daily basis for four weeks. They were then weighed, measured, and assessed for blood fats, sugars, and insulin levels. Researchers found that the group ingesting *Bifidobacteria breve* and *Lactobacillus acidophilus*, two types of probiotics found in many fermented foods, had significantly lower weight, abdominal measurements, blood sugar levels, triglycerides, and harmful as well as total cholesterol levels than the rats that didn't ingest the probiotics.[20]

In another study researchers fed rats a diet of salami, chocolate, chips, and biscuits — or, as they referred to it, the "cafeteria diet." As part of an obesity study conducted in Dordrecht, Netherlands, and published in the journal *Age*, researchers fattened the rats, some of whom were given probiotics while others were not. Scientists found that the probiotics were effective in preventing obesity because they had an anti-inflammatory effect.[21]

Ingesting foods rich in probiotics has been found to cause weight loss, the loss of back fat, and lowered levels of insulin, triglycerides, and other obesity indicators. In a study published in the *Journal of Applied Microbiology*, scientists found that the probiotic *Lactobacillus plantarum* lowered the levels of the various obesity indicators while also causing a reduction in overall weight, with a particular emphasis on back fat loss. They concluded that this probiotic has anti-obesity effects even in animals fed a high-fat diet and could be used in preventing and treating obesity.[22]

Many different strains of probiotics may be beneficial to your weight-loss efforts, but the *Lactobacillus* strains seem to be particularly valuable in this capacity. Fortunately, *Lactobacillus* bacteria are prevalent in most fermented foods and in most, if not all, of the recipes in this book. A Russian study published in the journal *Voprosy Pitaniia* found that adding yogurt fermented with live cultures of *Lactobacillus acidophilus* was effective for weight loss in overweight and obese individuals.[23]

Other research shows that probiotics improve insulin resistance in animals. In a study published in the *Chinese Journal of Contemporary Pediatrics*, scientists found that both *Lactobacillus acidophilus* and *Bifidobacterium breve* decrease blood fat and blood sugar levels and improve insulin resistance in animals, but *Bifidobacterium breve* was more effective at regulating insulin resistance than *L. acidophilus*, making it an important part of regulating insulin resistance, metabolic syndrome, or type 2 diabetes.[24]

In a pilot study of obese individuals with high blood pressure, researchers found that supplementing the diet with a probiotic-rich cheese improved the body mass index (BMI) and blood pressure, both of which are recognized markers of metabolic syndrome, and therefore shows additional promise for both metabolic syndrome and obesity.[25] The cheese used in the study was rich in the probiotic *Lactobacillus plantarum*, which is not normally found in most cheeses. However, I have included several recipes for delicious cheeses and, provided you use a probiotic supplement rich in *L. plantarum*, the cheese you make will also contain this obesity-reducing probiotic.

Many people think, "My grandparents were overweight, my parents are overweight, and I am overweight — it must be our genes." Although genes do play a role in most health conditions, that doesn't mean genetics are the primary factor. Even when genes are a factor, increasing amounts of research show that lifestyle factors like diet and exercise play a significant role in whether the genes for obesity — or any condition, for that matter — will turn off. The genes operate like light switches: just because a person may have genetic weaknesses or a predisposition to certain health conditions doesn't mean they will necessarily experience the health issue.

The burgeoning field of nutrigenomics studies the effects of food and nutrition on genetics, and scientists in this field increasingly agree that what you eat can determine whether the genes for particular health problems, including obesity, will "turn on."

Probiotic-rich foods also appear to play a role in the "turning on of genes," which is known in the scientific realm as *gene expression*. New research published in the *European Journal of Nutrition* found that certain *Lactobacilli* may reduce the likelihood of gene expression in fat tissue.[26] Although the research is still in the preliminary phase, the initial results spark excitement that beneficial bacteria may help determine whether our predisposition to certain health conditions, including obesity, are realized.

The new research into the connection between gut health, probiotics, and obesity offers hope and a novel potential treatment approach in the future. In a study published in *Beneficial Microbes*, scientists confirmed that altering specific gut bacteria could result in weight loss.[27]

As you can see, there is a rapidly growing body of research that supports the use of fermented foods to reset the body's metabolism and weight. It doesn't happen overnight, but trust in the body's natural ability to heal itself when given the right foods with the right health-supporting nutrients and probiotics within them. Of course, you can't simply eat fermented foods once a week or once a month and expect miracles, but if you give your body a variety of different fermented foods on a daily basis, you'll help restore your gut health. This will help reduce inflammation in your body, which will help improve your blood sugar levels and fire up your metabolism, all of which support healthy weight loss if you are overweight.

If you want to keep yourself healthy or improve your health, go with your gut. And the best way to go with your gut is to add fermented foods to your everyday diet.

More Health Benefits of Fermented Foods

You may have been shocked when I told you that approximately nine-tenths of your body's cells are actually bacteria and that an additional 100 trillion bacteria inhabit various parts of your body and play critical roles in your health. But don't let it scare you: after all, you could not live without these microorganisms, most of which ensure a healthy flora balance in your body. Most of these bacteria reside in your gut and play a significant role in your ability to lose weight or to maintain a healthy weight.

Probiotics are essential in ensuring the proper elimination of waste materials from the intestines, manufacturing important nutrients, controlling harmful bacteria and yeast populations, and many other necessary functions.

There are so many health benefits of eating fermented foods. Although I will go into further detail of the benefits of each fermented food in the relevant chapters, here is a basic overview of some more of the specific health rewards fermented foods offer:

Ten Ways Specific Fermented Foods Can Improve Your Life

1. Eating sauerkraut helps protect you from breast cancer. When cabbage is fermented as it is in making sauerkraut, its nutrients, known as glucosinolates, transform into the powerhouse anticancer nutrients isothiocyanates. Researchers have found that isothiocyanates balance excessive hormone production linked to breast cancer and even suppress tumor growth.[28]

2. Kimchi is the medicine of the future. Scientists have identified a whopping 970 different probiotic species in kimchi, many of which

offer powerful immune-boosting effects. Some of these unique probiotics are proven to kill superbugs even when our most potent medicines fail! The *Journal of Medicinal Food* found that kimchi's additional health properties include anticancer properties, anti-obesity benefits, anticonstipation, colorectal health promotion, cholesterol reduction, fibrolytic effect (a process that prevents blood clots from growing), antioxidative and anti-aging properties, brain health promotion, immune promotion, and skin health promotion.[29]

3. Regular consumption of miso fights at least five different types of cancer. Research published in multiple medical journals, including the *International Journal of Oncology*, found that miso consumption prevents and even effectively treats lung, liver, breast, colon, and liver cancers.[30]

4. Eating yogurt can reduce four markers essential for preventing diabetes and heart disease. Research published in the journal *Nutrition* demonstrated that yogurt cultured with the probiotic *L. plantarum* improved cholesterol levels, blood sugar balance, and homocysteine levels in women with metabolic syndrome.[31] As stated earlier (page 15), metabolic syndrome is a cluster of four symptoms, and when they occur together, they increase a person's risk of diabetes as well as heart disease and stroke. So reducing these markers bodes well for long-term health.

5. Eating certain fermented foods can alleviate seasonal allergies. Fermented plums contain beneficial yeasts known as *Saccharomyces cerevisiae* that have been linked to reducing allergies, congestion, and sinusitis. But why pop expensive supplements when you can reap these benefits and enjoy my Cultured Plum Chutney?

6. Eating fermented foods can give your brain a boost. Exciting new research published in the *Journal of Physiological Anthropology* found that intentionally boosting beneficial microbes by adding fermented foods to the diet could directly activate neural pathways between the gut and the brain and may boost brain health and prevent depression.[32]

7. Eating nondairy yogurt can improve bone density and reduce the risk of osteoporosis. Research published in the *International Journal*

of Food Science and Nutrition and multiple other journals found a direct link between dairy-free yogurt consumption and bone health.

8. Drinking probiotic-rich kefir helps protect against cancer and even effectively treats the disease. Kefir contains a probiotic called *Lactobacillus kefiri P-IF*, which is effective against leukemia even when multiple cancer drugs fail.

9. Eating fermented soy, known as miso, can prevent radiation injury. It's not just an urban myth: medical research conducted in Hiroshima found that eating fermented soy protects against the damaging effects of radiation — a growing concern in our modern society.[33]

10. Fermented foods are the missing link when it comes to effortless and permanent weight loss. In many studies the intestines of overweight and obese people were found to differ from those of lean people. Research published in the medical journal *Beneficial Microbes* found that obese and overweight people tend to have a higher ratio of harmful microbes to beneficial ones.[34] The best way to boost beneficial microbes to benefit from their slimming properties is to enjoy fermented foods that contain live cultures on a regular basis.

These health benefits are just the tip of the iceberg. New studies are being released on an almost daily basis, demonstrating the health benefits of incorporating more probiotics and probiotic-rich foods into the diet.

Throughout each of the upcoming chapters I'll share the health benefits of eating more probiotic-rich fermented foods. Soon you'll learn how easy it is to make more fermented foods at home. But first let's explore what happens in your gut, as it determines so much of the health throughout the rest of your body.

What Is a Microbiome?

Most of us consider ourselves to be individuals, not ecosystems, but we are so much more than just "us." Since the beginning of the Human Microbiome Project (HMP) — the microbial equivalent of cataloguing DNA in the Human Genome Project — researchers discovered that each human being is actually a vast ecosystem that is home to whole communities of microorganisms.[35] That's basically what scientists refer to when they talk about our *microbiome* — the various microorganisms that live in our mouth and nose and on our hands, wrists, knees, and so on. Every part of our body actually hosts a collection of microorganisms. So far the HMP has discovered that, like our fingerprints, no two microbiomes are exactly the same — yours is different from mine. Even your left hand differs from your right hand, and the fronts of your hands differ from the backs of your hands. At this point the cataloguing of the various bacteria continues. The trillions of bacteria inhabiting our bodies are a product of our life experience and are unique to each of us. Obviously, we are much more than just bacterial compilations, but the microbiome is an added dimension that few of us know about ourselves.

While the researchers are cataloguing the bacteria in multiple places on our bodies, the gut has been the focal point of their research, for good reason: what happens in your gut plays a significant role in determining the health of your whole body because your gut plays a critical role in the health of your brain, immune system, joints, respiratory system, skin, and much more. There are more microbes in your digestive tract than there are cells in your entire body.

It may sound creepy to think of the bacteria with whom you share your body, but you actually depend on most of them for your life. You literally could not live without many of these bacteria. Instead of being "creeped out" by them, feel grateful for the work they do to keep you healthy and alive. But it also means you need to pay greater attention to your gut health if you want to live a healthy, vibrant life.

Normally our gut has plentiful amounts of beneficial microbes along with some harmful ones we may have encountered along the way. Most of the time the beneficial microbes keep the harmful ones in check, but sometimes our dietary and lifestyle choices can wreak havoc on our gut health. Here are some of the main culprits that throw off our microbial balance.

Twenty Things That Throw Off the Microbial Balance in Our Gut

Our microbiome is like a complete ecosystem replete with trillions of beneficial bacteria and yeasts; however, it is also vulnerable to the overgrowth of harmful microorganisms such as pathogenic bacteria, fungi, and yeasts. Some of these pathogens can contribute to food poisoning, while others cause intestinal yeast infections, and still others can result in an excessively permeable gut (known as leaky gut syndrome) and inflammation anywhere in the body.

There are many factors that throw off the delicate microbial balance in our intestines. Here are the top twenty:

1. alcohol consumption
2. antacid use
3. antibiotic use
4. birth control pills
5. blood sugar imbalances
6. chlorinated water
7. consumption of antibiotic- and synthetic-hormone-containing foods
8. diabetes
9. excessive sugar intake
10. hypothyroid function
11. immune-suppressing drugs
12. inadequate hydrochloric acid production
13. mercury amalgam dental fillings
14. multiple sexual partners or sex with an affected person
15. nutritional deficiencies
16. poor diet
17. recreational drug use
18. stress, particularly chronic stress
19. toxic exposures
20. weakened immunity

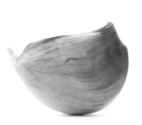
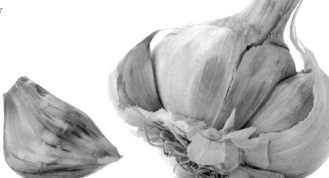

How to Heal Your Gut after Antibiotic Use

If you've ever taken a course of antibiotics, then you're probably familiar with some of the side effects of these drugs, including gastrointestinal distress, overgrowth of harmful bacteria in the intestines, and the resulting diarrhea. For many people the aftermath of taking antibiotics is as bad as the health problems that led them to take antibiotics in the first place.

That's because antibiotics indiscriminately kill bacteria in the intestines — good and bad. This is why so many people suffer from diarrhea while taking these drugs. The first step in healing your body after antibiotic use is to restore a healthy microbial balance. Antibiotics, although frequently helpful in killing harmful bacterial infections, also sway the overall gut bacterial balance by killing beneficial microbes. To help restore the microbial balance you'll want to increase the diversity of beneficial bacteria as well the numbers of specific probiotics.

The best way to improve the diversity of beneficial bacteria is to eat more fermented foods. Sorry, yogurt lovers: although yogurt can help boost the overall numbers of beneficial bacteria, it isn't great at improving the diversity of microbes, as it usually has only two to three strains of probiotics, if it contains live cultures at all. If you choose yogurt, avoid sweetened varieties because the sugar will also feed the harmful bacteria that are already overgrown. The best way to avoid excess amounts of sugar as well as ensure the viability of the probiotics in your yogurt is to make your own. (You'll find a simple recipe for making your own dairy-free yogurt on page 44.)

Some of the best fermented foods to boost bacterial diversity in your gut include kimchi, sauerkraut (not pasteurized varieties — choose types with live cultures in the refrigerator section of your local health food or grocery store), pickles (not the kind made with vinegar — choose naturally fermented options), and kombucha. Try to eat a small but increasing amount of fermented foods every day.

You may also benefit from a probiotic supplement, preferably one that contains strains of probiotics that have research-proven benefits against antibiotic-related symptoms, including *L. acidophilus, L. casei, L. plantarum, L. bulgaricus, L. reuteri,* and *S. thermophilus*.[36]

Research published in the *World Journal of Gastroenterology* also shows that the higher the dose of probiotics, the lower the incidence and duration of antibiotic-related symptoms like diarrhea.[37] Ideally it is best to take probiotic supplements and fermented foods prior to or at the start of a course of antibiotics, but if you are already taking antibiotics or still suffering from their effects even though you're no longer taking them, it is still a good idea to get started on probiotic-rich fermented foods.

Although diarrhea during or after antibiotic use may not seem like a big deal, it demonstrates the rampant destruction of important intestinal bacteria, which can set the stage for other health conditions. A growing number of health conditions, ranging from allergies to arthritis, have been linked to gut health, so restoring the integrity of the gut and its beneficial bacteria colonies and diversities is essential.

Boost Your Microbiome for Better Health

There are many ways to give your microbiome a boost, which in turn promises better health in the long term. Here are some simple things you can do to boost the health of your microbiome:

Eat probiotic-rich fermented foods daily, including kimchi, sauerkraut, and yogurt, to name a few. You'll discover many more in this book.

Eat a plant-based diet. That doesn't mean you need to give up meat entirely (unless, of course, you want to), but it does mean prioritizing plant-based foods in your diet, including vegetables, fruit, nuts, grains, beans, and seeds.

Reduce your sugar consumption. Harmful bacteria and yeasts feed on sugar and can quickly throw off the good-to-harmful balance of microbes in your gut.

Drink more water. Water is needed to ensure regular bowel movements and bowel health.

Eat plenty of high-fiber foods like legumes (chickpeas, pinto beans, kidney beans, black beans, etc.), seeds (flax, chia, hemp, sunflower, sesame, pumpkin, etc.), and whole grains (brown rice, millet, amaranth, or quinoa — look for sustainably grown, fair-trade options). Fiber helps keep the bowels moving and prevents stagnation.

What's the Difference Between Probiotics and Prebiotics?

But what about *prebiotics*? What's all the fuss about them? And are they really necessary for a healthy gut and a healthy body?

Like humans, probiotics need food to live. *Prebiotics* is a fancy word for the food that beneficial microbes need to survive. While many probiotic supplements include prebiotics in the form of fructooligosaccharides (FOS) or inulin, in my opinion these added prebiotics aren't necessary if you eat whole grains, fruits, legumes, or vegetables fairly regularly. More importantly, these ingredients may actually take up valuable space in a probiotic supplement that is better served by the probiotics themselves.

The addition of prebiotics to probiotic supplements is more of a marketing strategy than a health necessity. Although prebiotics do encourage the growth of probiotics, the truth is that if you're eating a diet high in fiber, along with fruit or fruit juices, vegetables, grains, and legumes, then you're probably getting all the prebiotics that beneficial bacteria need to thrive inside your gut anyway.

Prebiotics are essentially just natural carbohydrates in the form of sugars, starches, and fiber. They are found in almost any plant-based foods — I say "almost," but I can't think of one plant-based food that doesn't contain prebiotics.

Most people should be getting the food for probiotics (prebiotics) from their daily diet, and the fermented foods contained within this book naturally contain plentiful amounts of them. That's how the microbes transform fruits, vegetables, nuts, and seeds into the taste sensations we know as fermented foods.

Of course, outside of the fermented foods you enjoy, you should also make sure you enjoy a high-fiber diet on a regular basis, including vegetables, whole grains, and legumes (chickpeas, black beans, lentils, kidney beans, etc.).

If you're still concerned about boosting your dietary intake of prebiotics like inulin and FOS, the following are among the best sources of prebiotics you'll discover in *The Cultured Cook* and its recipes:

Fruits: apples, bananas, grapefruit, nectarines, peaches, pomegranate, and watermelon

Vegetables: asparagus, beets, cabbage, endive, fennel, garlic, Jerusalem artichokes, leeks, onions, peas, radicchio, shallots, snow peas

Legumes, nuts, and grains: black beans, cashews, chickpeas (garbanzo beans), kidney beans, lentils, oatmeal, oats, pinto beans, pistachios, soy milk, soybeans, tofu, and white beans

Incorporating more of these foods in your diet will significantly boost your number of health-boosting probiotics too. As you flip through the many recipes in *The Cultured Cook* you'll quickly see that many of these prebiotic foods can be found in the fermented foods themselves. That will help ensure not only the development of more probiotics during the culturing process but that you get more prebiotic foods to help multiply the numbers of any probiotics already in your intestines. And that will result in a healthier gut and a healthier you.

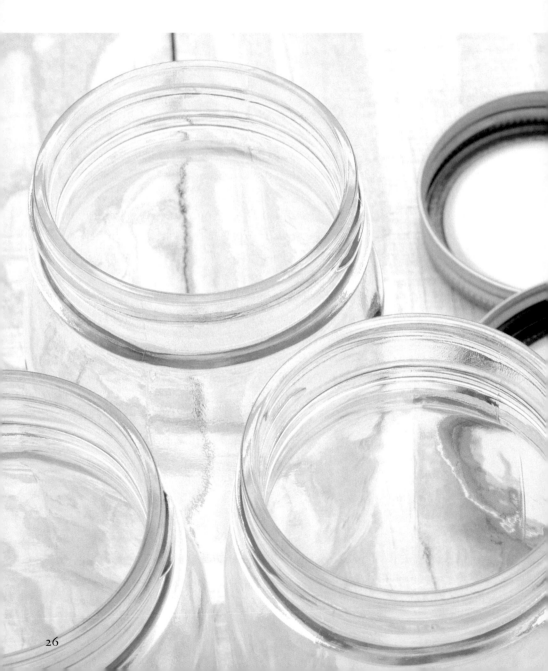

CHAPTER TWO

DAIRY-FREE YOGURT

Many years ago, when I was sixteen, a friend asked me if I wanted to try the Greek restaurant in downtown Hamilton, Ontario. Until that time I had only eaten Greek salad, which I loved, but I hardly considered it a full-blown Greek culinary repertoire. Being naturally adventurous with food, I immediately agreed to expand my horizons. I already had my driver's license and had saved up for my own car, albeit a junker straight out of the junk-yard (don't forget: I was sixteen and funds were limited), so I picked up my friend, and we headed downtown for our big, fat Greek adventure. We ate spanakopita (Greek spinach pastries made with paper-thin phyllo dough), a variety of black and green olives, Greek salad, freshly made pita breads, hummus, and tzatziki (a cucumber yogurt dip), and we ended the evening with pistachio baklava (Greek dessert pastries with nuts, honey, and phyllo) and yogurt drizzled with honey and walnuts. I loved every bite and was in-stantly hooked on Greek food.

While I had eaten store-bought yogurt, replete with fruit that more ac-curately resembled sugary jam on the bottom, I had never tasted tzatziki made from homemade yogurt or delighted in yogurt drizzled with honey and walnuts. I began buying Greek yogurt, which at the time was not the popular stuff it is now, so I had to shop around the city to find it. But when I did, I ate it almost every day with walnuts and honey. I still have fond memories of my Greek food extravaganza and the months of yogurt eating it inspired.

Years later I discovered that I was allergic to dairy products, so my yogurt-eating days came to a screeching halt. I went many years without eating any, but I still secretly longed for this delightful tart treat. So I began experimenting with plant-based yogurt options with the hope of finding one that was as good as the dairy versions but easy enough to make at home. It took a lot of experimentation, but I finally created dairy-free yogurt that was delicious and required almost no extra effort and no special or expensive equipment. I will share my yogurt-making innovations shortly, along with clear, step-by-step instructions in my recipes for World's Easiest Yogurt, Cultured Coconut Cream, and others. But first, let's explore the many health benefits of plant-based yogurt so you'll know exactly why you'll want to put forth the negligible effort to make your own.

In this chapter you'll discover easy and delicious recipes for:

- Traditional Vegan Yogurt
- World's Easiest Yogurt
- Cultured Coconut Cream
- Dairy-Free Cream

In Praise of Yogurt

Although today yogurt is perhaps the most widely known and eaten fermented food in North America and parts of Europe, the yogurt fad is not a new one. Humans have been obsessed with yogurt for thousands of years since it was first created or — perhaps more aptly — discovered.

The history of yogurt is an interesting one. The word *yogurt* is Turkish, but because this fermented creation is eaten in nations around the world and has been for so many years, its exact origin is unknown. Many people believe that the Babylonians started fermenting milk around 5000 BCE — a shocking seven thousand years ago — to create yogurt. Recent research has discovered a type of bacterial species known as *Lactobacillus delbrueckii bulgaricus*, which scientists believe originated on the surface of a plant. The bacteria are commonly used in making yogurt today due to their impressive ability to ferment milk or milk substitutes, thickening it and causing a separation of the thicker parts of the milk (curds) from the liquid part (whey). Therefore, milk may have become inadvertently inoculated by a nearby plant covered with these probiotic bacteria, resulting in fermented milk or, as we have come to call it, yogurt.

Yogurt appears in ancient Indian and Persian records, and the oldest written references to it are attributed to Pliny the Elder, who wrote that some "barbarous nations" could "thicken the milk into a substance with an agreeable acidity."[1]

Since then, yogurt has played an important role in the diets of Russian, Western Asian, and Southeastern and Central European people for centuries. Russian Nobel laureate and biologist Ilya Mechnikov believed that Bulgarian peasants' unusually long life spans were attributable to their regular consumption of yogurt. And I believe that Mechnikov may have been right, at least in part. More and more research on yogurt's health benefits indicates it may help in preventing and even treating many health conditions.

Some Serious Health Advantages of Regularly Eating Yogurt

Eating yogurt regularly has been found to reduce cholesterol and normalize blood sugar levels as well as reduce homocysteine levels, which will likely reduce the likelihood of experiencing the many diseases and health issues linked to high homocysteine levels, including Alzheimer's disease, diabetes, heart attack, and stroke.[2] Regular yogurt consumption has also been linked to a reduction in the duration of respiratory infections, an improvement in learning and memory, and even anticancer effects.[3] Keep in mind that these health advantages are based on the specific strains of probiotics found in the products tested, which varied significantly, so it is always a good idea to try different products periodically to obtain a greater variety of health-boosting strains. Better yet, make your own yogurt to ensure the viability and, therefore, health benefits of the live cultures found in it.

Here are some of the many ways yogurt gives your health a serious boost:

Preventing metabolic syndrome: Yogurt that contains live cultures of the probiotic strain *Lactobacillus plantarum* (not all yogurt contains this probiotic) has been shown to balance blood sugar, cholesterol, and homocysteine levels in women, all of which, when out of balance, are contributing factors for metabolic syndrome (see chapter 1, page 15). Metabolic syndrome is also characterized by excess abdominal fat and is often a precursor of other health conditions. To ensure you prevent metabolic syndrome through your yogurt consumption, check package labels to see if the yogurt you select contains live strains of *L. plantarum*, or better yet, make your own yogurt with *L. plantarum* starter cultures. I'll explain more about choosing your yogurt starter cultures on page 34. Although this study was specifically done on postmenopausal women, the results likely apply to premenopausal and menopausal women as well as men.

Treating respiratory infections: The probiotic strain *L. casei* found in most yogurts with live cultures has been shown to decrease the duration of respiratory infections as well as the severity of nasal congestion linked to infections.[4]

Improving gastrointestinal health: A study published in the *Journal of the American College of Nutrition* assessed the effects of consuming yogurt containing live *L. casei* cultures on common gastrointestinal infections in shift workers. The researchers found that yogurt consumption could reduce the risk of GI infections.[5]

Increasing nutrient Absorption: Consuming yogurt increases the quantity of nutrients absorbed from other foods eaten at the same meal, not just from the yogurt itself. A study in the *International Journal of Food Science and Nutrition* found that yogurt consumption increased the absorbability of the phytonutrients called isoflavones found in soy milk when the two foods were eaten at the same morning meal.[6] Of course, fermented soy or other dairy-free yogurt would likely have the same effect.

Preventing cancer: In preliminary animal studies, researchers found that eating yogurt that contains the probiotic *L. casei* has anticancer effects. Published in the medical journal *Immunobiology*, the research showed that *L. casei* worked on multiple levels: first, it blocked tumor development; second, it delayed its growth; third, it improved the body's immune response so that it could more effectively attack the tumor; and fourth, it reduced the number of blood vessels that fed the tumor.[7] The research was specifically conducted with breast cancer tumors in mice, making yogurt consumption a possible weapon against this deadly disease. Of course, more studies, including human ones, will give us greater insight into the benefits of *L. casei*, but considering the many health benefits and the lack of harmful side effects, it is worth giving yogurt some serious thought as part of an anticancer program.

Fighting *H. pylori* infections: While I mentioned the gastrointestinal health benefits of consuming yogurt, it also helps ward off the nasty *H. pylori* bacteria, which is increasingly joining the ranks of resistant superbugs. According to research published in the *World Journal of Gastroenterology*, yogurt consumption significantly helps to fight *H. pylori* infections, which have been linked to ulcers, gastritis, and cancer of the body's glandular and lymphatic tissues.[8]

Preventing food poisoning and colitis: Some strains of beneficial bacteria used during the fermentation process may actually help to prevent spoilage and reduce the likelihood of experiencing food poisoning. Yogurt fermented with the probiotic strain *L. paracasei* protected against salmonella infections and perhaps even the formation of colitis by inhibiting the body's release of inflammatory compounds while also increasing the release of anti-inflammatory compounds.[9]

Improving brain health: The last thing you probably think of when eating yogurt is how it may be helping your brain. But according to an animal study presented in the journal *Nutritional Neuroscience*, consuming whey, the clearish liquid by-product of yogurt production, can actually improve learning and memory.[10] Most types of yogurt, especially thinner varieties, tend to contain some residual whey. This is especially true of homemade yogurt.

You don't have to eat dairy yogurt to receive yogurt's many health benefits. There are many vegan alternatives to cow's milk yogurt, including coconut, cashew, almond, and soy (be sure to choose organic only, as soy is a heavily genetically modified crop). Don't be afraid to try to make these types of yogurt yourself. You'll find recipes in this book for cashew and almond yogurt, which can be easily adapted to other dairy-free options. Keep in mind that not all foods make great yogurt. I experimented with many different varieties over the years, and I can say without a doubt that navy bean yogurt is best left as a distant mishap in my kitchen — I did not include the recipe in this book.

Eight Tips to Buying Better Yogurt

While I am hoping to convey that making your own yogurt is simpler than you might think and that the added nutritional benefits far outweigh the effort, I realize that there are times when it might be easier to cheat by buying the store-bought varieties. After all, even the most diligent chefs sometimes purchase food items when they are in a pinch or feeling overworked, so on occasion you may wish to buy yogurt instead of making it yourself. Despite all the hype, not all the store-bought varieties of yogurt are good for you. Here are eight tips to help you select the best and healthiest store-bought yogurt for you:

1. Look for live cultures. Whichever kind of yogurt you purchase, make sure to check either on the ingredient list or somewhere on the package for "live cultures." These live cultures in yogurt provide the many beneficial gut and overall health benefits we attribute to yogurt. So find one that indicates that the yogurt has these live cultures.

2. Check the sugar content. Beware of hidden sugars that could sabotage the best efforts of the probiotics contained in yogurt. Check the number of grams of sugar along with the serving size to determine how much sugar you'll get if you eat the amount of yogurt you intend to eat. Some yogurt contains a whopping 26 to 29 grams of sugar for an individual serving of yogurt — that's more than many soft drinks or doughnuts. Most of the sugars naturally present in milk or milk alternatives should be eliminated during the culturing process because the sugars act as food for the probiotic cultures. If the yogurt contains much sugar, then either the manufacturer added sugar to the yogurt after the culturing process or the culturing process didn't take place and the manufacturer instead added flavors and thickening agents to the milk. Avoid any products with greater than 15 grams of sugar per serving, which is still fairly high and should be reserved as a treat rather than eaten on a regular basis.

3. Check the serving size. Some brands of yogurt list the amount of nutrients and sugars for a four-ounce serving, even though the container is six ounces, while others indicate a true six- or eight-ounce serving size. Be mindful of serving size so that you can compare the amount of protein, carbohydrates, and other nutrients based on equivalent serving sizes.

4. Avoid any yogurt that says it has been "heat treated" after the culturing process or during the packaging process. The beneficial probiotics that proliferate during the yogurt-making process are heat sensitive. If they are heated during packaging or at another stage of the manufacturing process, you will likely not reap any of the health benefits of eating the yogurt. These products are better left at the store.

5. Avoid yogurt with fillers. Making yogurt takes two ingredients: a type of milk or milk alternative and live cultures. The cultures do the work to transform the milk into yogurt. If the yogurt you purchase contains more ingredients than just milk and live cultures, it probably contains harmful ingredients like sugar, colors, fillers, or other less-than-healthy substances like carrageenan and xanthan gum. They are best avoided.

6. Go Greek. When it comes to yogurt varieties, Greek or plain yogurt are preferable because most of these varieties contain fewer ingredients and avoid colors, fillers, or sweeteners. Of course, you'll still want to check for live cultures and nasty ingredients — just because it is Greek doesn't mean that the manufacturer hasn't degraded the product.

7. Look for dairy-free yogurt alternatives. In my research I found that dairy-free yogurt varieties often contain a greater diversity of probiotic strains than dairy yogurt. That doesn't mean all dairy-free yogurt is better than cow's milk yogurt, but it does mean that if you're vegan or just avoiding milk products, you can still reap yogurt's health benefits.

8. Choose organic as much as possible if you're choosing cow's milk yogurt. Cow's milk frequently contains antibiotic or other medication residues as well as the genetically modified hormone known as rBST. BST is a hormone known as bovine somatotropin; rBST is a genetically modified version of BST that Monsanto developed by using genetically engineered *E. coli* bacteria. It is probably not something you want in your body.

Of course, there are no hard and fast rules about choosing the best commercial variety of yogurt, particularly as there are many manufacturing and processing variables that determine the quality of the yogurt. But the above guidelines will help you select the best one for your buck.

The Essentials of Making Probiotic-Rich Yogurt

Commercial yogurt simply cannot compare to homemade yogurt, and not just because of the taste and purity of ingredients but also because of the health benefits. Homemade yogurt tends to contain more live probiotic cultures, while many commercial varieties do not. Here are the things you'll want to consider before making your own yogurt:

Starter Cultures

One of the essential elements of making yogurt is to ensure you have a good starter culture — the beneficial bacteria that significantly multiply during the fermentation process, resulting in the separation of curds and whey. You have a few options. First, you can choose a product that is specifically marketed as "yogurt starter" or "yogurt starter culture." They can be a bit hard to find, and most are made from dairy-based yogurt and may not be suitable for people who are intolerant of or allergic to dairy products. Be sure to check the package to determine the source of the cultures. If the source is free of dairy products, it will say so on the package, but if it is from dairy products, it usually won't.

Second, you can purchase a probiotic supplement and use this for your yogurt starter cultures. Probiotic supplements come in capsule or powder form. You can choose either option. If you are vegan or intolerant of or allergic to dairy products, be sure to choose a supplement that is dairy-free, which should be listed on the label. Be sure the product you choose contains a variety of *Lactobacilli* bacteria, as these are the ones that do the work of turning the milk of your choice into yogurt. The product you choose may also contain various strains of *Bifidobacteria*, which are fine. Avoid any products that contain *S. cerevisae*, *S. salivarius*, or *S. boulardii* (basically, any of the probiotics that start with *S.*). Although these probiotics may have beneficial health effects, I have found that they add a less-than-desirable yeasty flavor to yogurt and are best avoided for the purposes of my recipes.

If you choose capsules, you'll simply empty the contents of the capsule into the recipe you're making according to the instructions. One standard-size capsule equals one-quarter teaspoon probiotic powder. If you're using small or large capsules, you may want to empty the contents into a quarter teaspoon to see whether it contains more or less than the amount called for in the recipes. For example, I often use capsules that are quite tiny and simply use the contents of two whenever I would normally use one. You may also find capsules that seem larger than normal, so measuring the contents to determine the size by volume can be helpful. Ultimately the amount of probiotics used in the recipes that follow doesn't need to be completely precise. Simply taste the yogurt (or cheese, as is the case in the next chapter if you're using probiotic capsules or powder as a starter culture) to determine whether it has reached the desired level of tanginess.

Higher amounts of probiotic powder (or higher amounts of the contents of probiotic capsules) tend to result in faster culturing times and tangier yogurt. As long as the probiotic powder or capsules you choose actually contain live probiotics, the recipes will work fine. Once you have emptied the capsule contents, you can discard the empty capsules. (I save them and use them for ingesting therapeutic essential oils, but that's a story for another book.) If you choose a powdered form of probiotics, simply use one-quarter teaspoon as the equivalent of one capsule.

Although in theory higher amounts of probiotics in the powder or capsules are better than lower amounts, it rarely works out so neatly in real life. For example, many companies claim there are 4 billion or 10 billion or some other number of probiotics in their product, but it doesn't actually contain the amount on the label. Some labels state these numbers "as of the time of packaging," while others state them "as of the expiration date," which is a huge difference. It is preferable to choose probiotics that state the amount as of the expiration date, as probiotic cultures tend to deteriorate and reduce in numbers from the time they are packaged. Ultimately there is only one good way to test the viability and quality of your cultures — make them into yogurt. If you get the tangy taste of yogurt or the milk separates into curds and whey, you'll know your probiotics worked and were, therefore, alive. In other words, don't get hung up on the marketing claims of higher numbers being superior. One of my favorite probiotic products contains tiny capsules of 4 billion probiotics each. I've tried some larger capsules with 10 or more billion probiotics, but I found that many are not as active at culturing yogurt. Choosing good yogurt cultures is not a numbers game, so don't spend too much time on that.

Containers and Utensils

You'll want to use only glass or ceramic bowls, dishes, or spoons for yogurt making, as probiotic cultures don't survive well when exposed to metals. I'd also avoid plastic because as yogurt forms, lactic acids likewise form, which can break down plastic. You definitely don't want plastic residue in your finished yogurt.

Fermentation and Temperature

After you've combined your dairy-free milk and probiotic starter cultures you'll want to let it sit undisturbed in a warm location — ideally between 110 and 115 degrees Fahrenheit or 43 and 46 degrees Celsius. Again, don't get too hung up on finding the perfect temperature. I've made successful batches of yogurt at room temperature; it just takes a bit longer for it to culture sufficiently to separate. You can place it in front of a heater (but not somewhere too hot, or else the heat will kill probiotic cultures), in the oven with just the pilot light on, or in a warm spot in your kitchen. After your yogurt has cultured, you'll notice it has separated into curds (the thick part) and whey (the clearish-yellowish liquid). You'll want to carefully spoon out the thick yogurt prior to refrigerating it or even moving it, because it quickly starts to mix, which makes it more difficult to spoon out the thick yogurt. After you've spooned off the thick yogurt, store it in a sealed glass bowl in the refrigerator for about a week.

Keep in mind that the separation of curds and whey only occurs when you're making yogurt in the traditional sense. I've innovated a new technique that has all the health benefits of yogurt with far less work and mess.

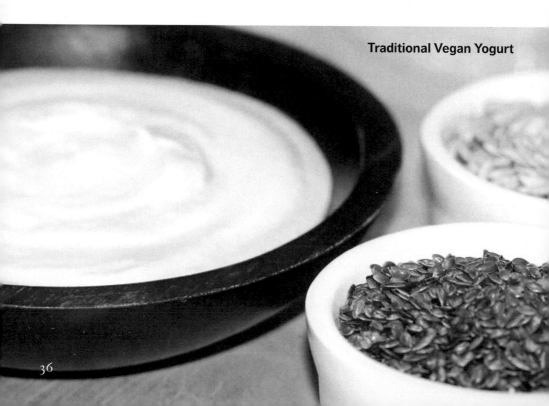

Traditional Vegan Yogurt

Traditional Vegan Yogurt

Making your own yogurt may seem daunting, but it is actually simple. Traditional methods involve heating the milk, but this yogurt is a vegan alternative. Save the whey, as it can be added to dips, dressings, smoothies, and other foods to give them beneficial probiotics, or use it as a starter culture for many other recipes: just add two tablespoons to any food you'd like to ferment, and the whey will initiate the fermentation process. The whey lasts about one week when stored in a covered jar in the fridge. Don't worry about the sweetener in the recipe, as it acts as prebiotics for the beneficial microbes, activating them to create yogurt; very little sugar is left in the final yogurt.

Makes about 2 to 2½ cups

2 cups raw, unsalted cashews
3 cups filtered water
1 teaspoon pure maple syrup or agave nectar
2 probiotic capsules or ½ teaspoon probiotic powder

Blend the cashews, water, and syrup or nectar until smooth. Pour into a medium saucepan, and heat over low heat until warm but not hot. Once it is lukewarm, pour the cashew milk into a clean, nonmetallic container such as a glass bowl or ceramic crock. (Metal containers can inhibit the culturing process.)

Add the contents of the probiotic capsules (discarding the empty capsule shells) or probiotic powder to the cashew milk. Stir the ingredients together until combined.

Cover the container, and let it sit undisturbed in a warm setting for eight to ten hours, or more if you prefer a tangier yogurt. Scoop out the thickened yogurt, and reserve the whey for another use.

Seven Myths about Yogurt

Myths about yogurt and probiotics abound. While conducting my research for this book, I was surprised to learn what many people are saying about yogurt. To help dispel misinformation, here are the seven most common myths about yogurt you need to be aware of. Keep in mind that it's not my intention to bash yogurt — after all, eating yogurt provides many health benefits. Rather, it is my goal to present it in an accurate light.

Myth 1: All yogurt is healthy. Not all yogurt is healthy. In fact, some is downright disgusting and contains more sugar than you'll find in doughnuts. And some yogurt is full of additives, colors, and gums (like xanthan gum or carrageenan) to thicken it and are best avoided altogether.

Myth 2: All yogurt contains beneficial probiotics. Many yogurts are heated during the manufacturing or shipping process and no longer contain the live cultures they boast on the label. Unfortunately, there is no easy way to find out whether the yogurt you buy contains live cultures other than to take a heaping tablespoon of it, add it to warmed milk or milk substitute, and leave it to rest for eight to ten hours. If you have a new batch of yogurt from your experiment, then you know the original yogurt you purchased contains live cultures. Otherwise it probably doesn't.

Myth 3: Yogurt is the best source of probiotics. Not even close. Don't get me wrong: unsweetened yogurt with live cultures is healthy and a great addition to any diet, but it isn't the best source of probiotics, not by a long shot. There's sauerkraut, kimchi, fermented pickles, curtido, kefir, and miso, to name a few — all of which tend to be higher in probiotics and contain many more varied strains of those good microbes than yogurt.

Myth 4: Yogurt contains a vast array of probiotic strains. Yogurt usually contains two or three different strains of probiotics, depending on the cultures used to inoculate the particular yogurt you're buying. Those strains are usually *Lactobacillus acidophilus*, *Lactobacillus bulgaricus*, and occasionally *Streptococcus salivarius* or Bifidobacteria. (Don't worry: there's no connection between *S. salivarius* and the strep bacteria that make you sick.)

Myth 5: Even people who are lactose intolerant or allergic to dairy products can eat yogurt. Because the cultures turn the milk sugar lactose into lactic acid, some people who are lactose intolerant can eat yogurt without digestive distress. Depending on the amount of lactose present in the end product (which is usually determined by the fermentation time and the activity of the particular cultures used), a person with a lactose intolerance may not be able to eat dairy-based yogurt. Additionally, anyone with a full-blown allergy to dairy products will still have an immune response to dairy yogurt and will need to avoid it altogether. Having said that, there are many excellent nondairy alternatives that still confer the health benefits of eating yogurt.

Myth 6: "I eat yogurt, so I get all the probiotics I need." I regularly hear this from people who consider themselves knowledgeable about health and wellness. They (incorrectly) believe that yogurt is a cure-all for what ails them and can correct any imbalances in their intestines. Because most yogurts contain only two or three strains of probiotics (out of the thousand or so currently known probiotics possible in our food), you're only going to reap the health benefits of taking those particular strains. However, the few strains found in yogurt offer many benefits, including easing traveler's diarrhea, boosting nutrient absorption, and treating *H. pylori* infections or food poisoning.

Myth 7: Dairy-based yogurts are nutritionally superior to nondairy-based yogurts. Although the amount of research assessing nondairy yogurts is still relatively small in comparison to dairy yogurt, there are some good studies showing the health benefits of the dairy-free versions. Dairy-free yogurt has been linked to reducing cholesterol levels and heart-disease markers as well as increasing anticancer activity.[11]

Even when yogurt is portrayed accurately, without embellishing its healing properties, this delicious food still warrants superfood status.

Nine Reasons to Ditch Dairy

While many people cite the health benefits of dairy-based yogurt, I do not include dairy products in my diet for a variety of reasons, most especially because I'm allergic to it. But even if you aren't allergic to dairy products, there are other reasons to nix dairy. Obviously some of the following reasons may be rectified by simply choosing organic milk or dairy products from cows or goats that are sustainably and ethically raised, but other issues are not so easily resolved. Here are some of the problems with commercially available dairy products.

1. **Cow's milk was intended for baby cows.** Baby cows have four stomachs in which to digest the proteins found in milk, which we humans don't have. We have one stomach, and it simply does not do the job of four.

2. **Most cows are fed commercial feed that simply should not be part of the food supply.** We are what we eat and what we eat eats! Much of the food fed to cows includes animal by-products, genetically modified soy, genetically modified corn, cottonseed, pesticides, antibiotics, and even chicken manure. These ingredients can then find their way into the substandard milk and dairy products sold in many stores.

3. **Dairy products contain hormones that are much stronger than human hormones.** By drinking milk or eating dairy products we are exposed to the hormones routinely given to plump up cows and increase milk production. Because our human hormonal balance is delicate, it is easily thrown off by drinking or eating dairy products that contain much stronger hormones than our own.

4. **Dairy products are mucus forming and can contribute to ear and sinus infections.** Whenever I've asked one of my clients to stop eating dairy products to resolve their ear and sinus problems, they unfailingly experience tremendous improvements in these conditions.

5. **Dairy does not offer easily digestible calcium.** "But how will I get my calcium?" you may be asking. I have heard this question countless times over twenty-five years of practicing and writing about health issues. You'd be surprised to learn that dairy marketing boards have conditioned us to equate milk and dairy products with calcium, but the truth is that humans do not easily digest the calcium in dairy products (as I mentioned above), and therefore it is not readily absorbed. Research even shows that the countries whose citizens consume the highest amounts of dairy products actually have the highest incidence of osteoporosis! Milk does the body good? Not when it comes to bone health.

6. **Milk is hard to digest.** Most milk is homogenized, which is a process that involves denaturing the proteins found in milk, making them even more difficult to digest than they originally were. Many people have immune system reactions to these denatured proteins. I believe homogenization and the resulting immune system reactions play a role in the growing incidence of allergies and autoimmune conditions.

7. Most dairy products are pasteurized to kill bacteria. While this process may be intended to destroy harmful, disease-causing bacteria, it also kills good bacteria and enzymes that are needed to ensure healthy gut health and digestion of the dairy products themselves. This pasteurization further strains our digestive processes and, specifically, the difficulty a growing number of people have digesting dairy products.

8. Health-harming pesticides find their way into the dairy products produced by cows due to the high amounts used in the farming of foods used for cow feed. Some of these pesticides have been linked to cancer or are considered neurotoxins (toxic compounds that harm the brain and nervous system). They are best avoided as much as possible.

9. Studies have linked dairy products to arthritis. Some researchers even use dairy products in animals' feed to produce joint inflammation consistent with arthritis.

There are many reasons to avoid dairy products altogether. While the live bacteria found in yogurt made from cow's milk can offer many health benefits, it doesn't offset all the inherent problems with dairy or the commercial production processes. Fortunately there are many excellent plant-based yogurt options to choose from, including almond, rice, cashew, oat, coconut, and possibly others.

How to Speed Up the Culturing Time of Yogurt

After making my first batch of World's Easiest Yogurt, I wanted it on a regular basis. And sometimes I craved it so much that I didn't want to wait overnight or eight to ten hours for it to ferment. The mad scientist in me set to work to find ways to speed up the yogurt-making process, and I am happy to report that my efforts were a success. I found multiple ways to get probiotics to work faster. That may make me sound like some kind of bacteria slave driver, but I amply rewarded them for their efforts. And when I combined all these newfound techniques, I got the fastest yogurt yet.

First, make sure you maintain a warm environment for the full culturing time. Ideally 110 to 115 degrees Fahrenheit or 43 to 46 degrees Celsius works, but any warm (but not hot) space is fine. I created a "warming station" using a small plastic heating pad for maintaining a steady temperature when making kombucha. I placed my glass or ceramic container of yogurt ingredients on this warming station and found that it definitely sped up the formation of bacterial cultures and that signature yogurt taste. It is not necessary to buy a special heating pad for this purpose, however. You can simply place your yogurt in the oven with the pilot light on or keep it in a warm spot in your kitchen or in front of a heater. I haven't tried using a traditional heating pad, but that might also work (be careful not to spill liquid onto the electrical components, as it could be a fire hazard). Alternatively, you can also heat a slow cooker filled with yogurt ingredients to 115 degrees Fahrenheit and then turn it off. Or you can use a crock from a slow cooker, warm it and the yogurt ingredients to 115 degrees Fahrenheit, turn it off, and remove the crock from the heating element and wrap in a towel to help retain the heat. Do not heat the ingredients in a microwave, as the microwaves destroy the probiotic cultures. You can also put the ingredients in a dehydrator with some of the shelves removed and set it to 100 degrees Fahrenheit (43 degrees Celsius).

Second, if you are using probiotic powder or capsules, double up on the amount used. This will help the probiotic bacteria increase their numbers faster, which in turn results in attaining yogurt's unique flavor faster as well. I have found that it reduces the fermentation time by approximately two hours in a recipe that requires eight to ten hours of fermentation time. Of course, there are other factors such as temperature, heat consistency, sugar content (as it provides the food for the probiotics), among others.

Third, add a small amount (one teaspoon to one tablespoon) of a natural sweetener, such as agave nectar, coconut nectar, honey, or pure maple syrup (not maple-flavored syrup, which is actually mostly corn syrup). These natural sweeteners fuel the growth of probiotics, which in turn speeds up yogurt-culturing time. Depending on how much sweetener you use and how long you leave your yogurt to culture, there will actually be few sugar molecules left in the final yogurt because the probiotics will eat them and use that energy for their growth. Avoid using artificial sweeteners like aspartame (Neotame), saccharin (Sweet'N Low), or sucralose (Splenda), as these sweeteners cannot serve as food for probiotics. Also, while stevia is a natural herbal sweetener, it doesn't have any sugar molecules, so it cannot feed probiotics. You can use stevia to sweeten yogurt after it has been made, to suit your taste preferences, but it will not help yogurt cultures grow.

Cultured Coconut Cream

Cultured coconut cream is a delicious, probiotic-rich cream that is the perfect replacement for dairy whipped cream. It contains all the benefits of coconut milk, including its medium-chain triglycerides, which have been found to help with weight loss, thyroid imbalances, and other health issues. Enjoy this delicious creamy treat with pancakes, waffles, fruit salad, or other dishes. Alternatively, use it as a sweet dip for fruit slices or atop a bowl of fresh berries.

Makes about 1 cup

One 14-ounce can coconut milk (regular coconut milk, not the "light" or low-fat versions)
1 probiotic capsule or ¼ teaspoon probiotic powder

In a small glass or ceramic bowl with a lid, empty the can of coconut milk. (Do not use a metal bowl, as metal can inhibit the culturing process.) If the cream and water have separated, mix them together.

Stir in the contents of the probiotic capsule (discarding the empty capsule shell) or the probiotic powder. Cover the bowl with a clean cloth, and leave in an undisturbed, warm setting for eight to ten hours. Remove the cloth, cover the bowl with a lid, and refrigerate.

After the mixture has cooled for at least an hour, the coconut cream is ready for use. The mixture will have separated during the culturing/cooling process, and the coconut cream is the thick top layer. Scoop out the cream, and either use it immediately or transfer it to another lidded glass container and store it in the refrigerator until you're ready to use it. The thinner liquid below the cream can be saved and added to smoothies and juices or used as a "starter" to culture other foods. The cream and starter liquid will last for about one week in the fridge.

World's Easiest Yogurt

One day, while I was busy straining whey from a batch of homemade dairy-free yogurt and waiting for what seemed like way too long, I said to myself, "There must be a better way." I knew that yogurt had been made this way for hundreds, perhaps thousands, of years, but that was when yogurt was made from only cow's, goat's, or camel's milk. While substituting cashews in place of milk, I set to work to find a better, no-muss, no-fuss method for making dairy-free yogurt. Realizing that the culturing time can only be sped up so much — after all, those little beneficial bacteria need time to work their magic — I also figured out that the best way to improve yogurt making was to remove the straining-curds-from-whey process, which is not only time-consuming and somewhat labor-intensive but also very messy. After a few tries I discovered that it *is* possible to make delicious, cultured yogurt without all the muss or fuss of straining curds from whey. While it still takes several hours for the probiotics to proliferate, giving yogurt its signature tangy taste, in a mere few minutes of actual prep time you can make your own yogurt. And, of course, you can set the probiotics to work while you sleep, thereby greatly reducing the seeming wait time for your fresh yogurt. Not only is this yogurt delicious, but it also tends to result in a larger diversity of probiotic strains than commercial yogurt...and you'll know from the taste whether it actually contains live cultures, which is hard to know when eating commercial varieties. Additionally, this recipe contains the fiber that is naturally found in the cashews (most unflavored yogurt contains none) and is naturally thick like Greek yogurt. And it thickens up even more when left to culture overnight, making the perfect base for sauces, salad dressings, and marinades. While perfecting this recipe, which I am thrilled to share with you here, I also discovered some ways to speed up the culturing process, described in detail on page 41.

Makes about 1 quart/liter

3 cups raw, unsalted cashews
2 cups filtered water
1 probiotic capsule or ¼ teaspoon probiotic powder
Pomegranate arils (seeds) or pitted frozen or fresh cherries for garnish (optional)

In a medium glass or ceramic bowl with a lid, combine the cashews with the water, and pour in the contents of the probiotic capsule (discarding the empty capsule shell) or the probiotic powder. Stir the ingredients together until combined.

Attach the lid, and let sit for eight to twenty-four hours, depending on how tangy you like your yogurt.

Puree the ingredients in a blender until smooth, then return the yogurt to the bowl. Garnish with pomegranate arils or cherries if desired, and enjoy immediately, or refrigerate for up to four days.

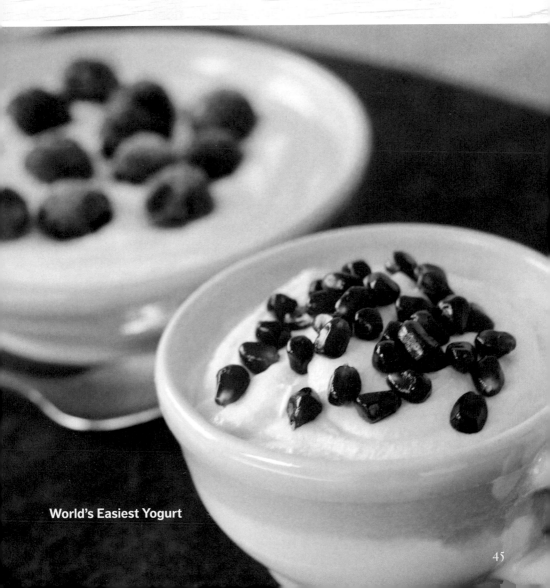

World's Easiest Yogurt

Dairy-Free Cream

Much like yogurt, this dairy-free cream is thick and smooth. But this cream tastes sweeter than yogurt, which is tart. You can use this dairy-free cream alongside baked goods, over fruit for a delicious and nutritious probiotic-rich dessert, or atop a hot chocolate. Keep in mind that if you use the cream in hot chocolate, the longer it is in contact with heat, the more probiotics are destroyed; most strains of probiotics cannot withstand much heat.

Makes about 1½ cups

½ cup almond milk
1 cup raw, unsalted cashews
2 fresh Medjool dates, pitted and coarsely chopped
2 probiotic capsules or ½ teaspoon probiotic powder

In a glass or ceramic bowl with a lid, combine the almond milk, cashews, and date pieces. Add the contents of the probiotic capsule (discarding the empty capsule shell) or the probiotic powder, and stir into the cashew mixture.

Cover the bowl, and let it sit in a warm, undisturbed setting for eight to ten hours or until you achieve your desired tanginess.

Blend the ingredients together until they are smooth, adding a small amount of water as necessary to enable blending. Serve immediately or refrigerate for up to one week.

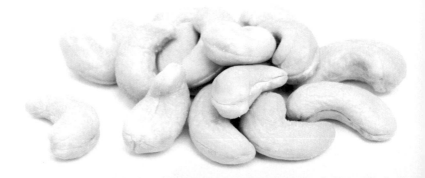

CHAPTER THREE

VEGAN CHEESES

I love cheese. I love the savory, salty flavors and the creamy textures. I love how cheese pairs with a diverse variety of foods, from fruit, to crackers and breads, to vegetable crudités and antipasto. I am far more likely to crave cheese than any other food. But I don't love how cheese makes me feel — at least not the standard variety of dairy cheeses. I am not only lactose intolerant (unable to digest milk sugar) but also fully allergic to dairy products. Sadly, that includes cheese. Even medical skin prick tests show my allergy to dairy products, which rarely occurs with food allergies.

As a nutritionist and doctor of natural medicine, I used to take comfort in the knowledge that most dairy products are not healthy options for a wide variety of reasons (check out the "Nine Reasons to Ditch Dairy" on page 40), but when I began to apply the fermentation techniques I learned over the years to nuts and seeds, I realized I could create delicious, creamy, and versatile cheeses and even cheesecakes completely free of dairy products. I saw that I don't have to live without cheese; I just need to focus my attention and diet on plant-based options, which are many and offer a wealth of unique and amazing flavors to draw from. Excited by my new discovery, I began experimenting with cheeses made from almonds, Brazil nuts, cashews, hazelnuts, macadamia nuts, pecans, pumpkin seeds, and sunflower seeds. I explored the addition of herbs, specific probiotic cultures, smoked salt, and other flavor enhancers. Then I began aging my cheeses, which helped them to develop sharper flavors, harder textures, and even the rinds that most of us expect only on dairy cheeses. Whereas many commercially available dairy cheeses contribute to negative health issues, even for those who can consume them, these plant-based cheeses include a wide variety of health-boosting probiotics — in other words, not only will you avoid the problems linked to eating dairy products, but you'll also give your health a big boost too. And unlike many of the rubbery faux cheeses on the market, these cheeses have silkier textures and a wider range of flavors to suit even the most discriminating palates.

In this chapter I'll introduce you to a world of cultured artisanal cheeses and their varying flavors. I'll present the basic cheese culturing processes as well as techniques for aging your cheeses to give them more distinct flavors, a wider range of textures, and unique appearances. The recipes you'll find in this chapter are:

- Gluten-Free, Dairy-Free Rejuvelac
- World's Easiest Yogurt Cheese
- Almond Farmer's Cheese
- Walnut Thyme Cheese
- Bracotta Cheese
- Chèvrew
- Macadamia Cream Cheese
- Aged Smoked Cheese
- Aged Miso Cheese
- Aged Savorella Cheese

How Traditional Dairy Cheeses Are Made

Although I will show you many cheese-making techniques that simplify the process of making plant-based cheeses, it is also important to understand how traditional cheese is made. Most dairy-based cheeses are made by heating the milk to kill all microbes and adding an acidifying compound to cause the milk to separate into curds and whey. The curds are the solid part of the curdled milk, and the whey is a clear yellowish liquid that has separated from it. The curds are then strained from the whey and then weighted down to draw out any excess moisture. Then, depending on the type of cheese being made, varying ingredients are added to build up a rind. Salt is the most commonly used ingredient because it draws out additional moisture while it also acts as a preservative to prevent harmful microbes from growing on the cheese. Additionally, depending on the type of cheese, different yeasts or other microbes are inoculated into the cheese to encourage their growth; these help the cheese obtain different flavors, colors, and textures. Of course, there are many variations to every aspect of this process, and some cheeses are made entirely differently.

Industrial processes have largely changed the way many cheeses are made, opting for sterilization, standardization, and commercialization over microbial variation, wild cultures, and artisanal cheeses. But there are still some cheese-making artists who work to keep the traditional processes and the quality cheeses they produce alive and well.

You may be wondering why I would bother discussing how dairy cheeses are made in a book that only includes recipes for nondairy cheeses. I want you to have a basic understanding of the traditional approach many cheese-makers have begun applying to plant-based cheeses. Nondairy cheesemakers follow essentially the same processes as traditional cheesemakers, but they make a "milk" from nuts, seeds, legumes, or grains. For example, a nondairy cheesemaker may first make a dairy-free milk from cashews or almonds be-fore following the remaining processes of traditional cheese making. While I think this process yields some impressive cheeses, in my recipes I sought ways to boost the nutritional and probiotic value of the cheeses. Addition-ally, like many of my readers, I often feel like there just aren't enough hours in a day: between writing books, blogs, magazine articles, conducting inter-views, and engaging my readers online, my schedule (and energy at the end of a busy work day!) rarely permits making vegan milks, straining off the fiber, then straining curds from whey, weighting them, and so on. So I found ways to achieve amazing artisanal plant-based cheeses without the labor-intensive processes of traditional methods.

I've worked for many years to find new ways to create cheeses that are nutritionally superior, take less effort, make less mess, and still have the amazing taste and textural nuances of other types of cheeses, whether dairy or plant based. I found that not only was it redundant to add water to nuts, seeds, or other food items and then to cook the milks with an acid to separate the food from the water, but also that many water-soluble or heat-sensitive nutrients like enzymes, B-complex vitamins, or vitamin C are destroyed during this process. And when you consider the time it takes to execute these processes as well as the clean-up time for all the pots, strainers, and other dishes involved, I decided it was a serious waste of valuable time.

You'll notice that I haven't tried to re-create dairy cheeses. You won't find any recipes for fake mozzarella, provolone, or Swiss cheese that inevitably taste nothing like the real thing. The truth is that plant-based cheeses taste different from their dairy counterparts. When people name them after dairy cheeses, the result is often disappointed cooks who thought they'd get something identical to Brie, mozzarella, or some other traditional cheese. That's not to say that the flavors of the vegan cheeses are inferior — they aren't, at least not when they are made using cultured techniques. They're simply different. Additionally, each of the vegan cheeses I have included here for you have unique and delightful flavor and texture nuances that differ from any other cheese. The various microbial cultures, combined with the techniques I've developed, result in cheeses that are works of food art in their own right and not mere copycats of dairy varieties. Or, as one of my friends says, "They are little pieces of heaven." In the same way that Brie is different from Roquefort and blue cheese is different from feta, so too are the variations among plant-based cheeses made from walnuts, cashews, Brazil nuts, or other ingredients.

I have tried many different nuts and seeds to use as the basis of my cheeses, including Brazil nuts, cashews, hazelnuts, pecans, sunflower seeds, and walnuts. Each one provides a different flavor and texture from the others. I also use a wide variety of natural, probiotic-rich ingredients to inoculate my cheeses with the cultures they need to age and to help their flavors develop, including rejuvelac (an enzyme- and probiotic-rich water made from soaking grains), yogurt, probiotic capsules or powders, miso (aged beans or rice), and sauerkraut or pickle brine.

Although many cheesemakers insist on wild cultures, in my experience the novice cheesemaker sometimes finds the spontaneous growth of a variety of molds a bit unnerving. Other cheesemakers insist on using only one strain of packaged yeast or bacterial cultures, but I believe the natural diversity from the above-mentioned starter cultures adds to the taste as well as the many health benefits of eating these cheeses. Of course, if you are inclined to delve into the art of cheese making by using wild strains of microbes, enjoy the experience.

Ultimately, while many people have forgotten that the primary purpose of eating is to nourish our cells and to rebuild our energy, the reality is that we need to replenish ourselves daily with the nutrients and microbial cultures needed to grow new and healthy cells, which form new and healthy tissue, which further forms new and healthy organs and organ systems.

I believe we can eat nourishing, healthful food that is absolutely delicious and no less satisfying than the less-healthy options many of us choose to eat for taste alone. The narrative that we must choose between healthy food and delicious food is false. We really can have our (healthier) cake and eat it too — or, in this case, our healthier cheesecake and eat it too.

Common Cheese-Making Ingredients to Avoid Like the Plague

You'll notice that none of these cheeses use any of the additives commonly used in many plant-based cheese recipes, such as carrageenan and xanthan gum. That's because these are unhealthy additives that contribute to many health problems.

Carrageenan: The Hidden Cheese Ingredient Linked to Pain and Inflammation

Carrageenan is a food additive that acts as a thickener or emulsifier, and it is so ubiquitous in the food industry that it is found in most packaged cheeses and other foods, restaurant sauces, and even many foods that have been certified organic. Carrageenan is even recommended in many vegan cheese-making books and for commercial plant-based cheese alternatives. Its origins seem harmless enough: it is derived from the seaweed known as Irish moss and is then processed to extract the ingredient.

Like most people, I originally thought carrageenan was just a seaweed extract, so I didn't give the question of whether it was healthy much consideration. Then I heard that researchers were giving animals carrageenan to induce pain and inflammation to prepare the animals for scientific studies exploring antipain drugs. So I began to investigate.

Dr. Joanne Tobacman has conducted many studies on the effects of carrageenan consumption, including a recent one published in the *Journal of Diabetes Research*.[1] After being fed carrageenan for only six days, animals developed glucose intolerance, an umbrella term used to describe impaired metabolism involving excessively high blood sugar levels. Dr. Tobacman found that the food additive caused blood sugar levels to skyrocket, and these results indicate that consuming carrageenan may lead to the development of diabetes. She states that because the carrageenan used in animals' diets so commonly causes diabetes, the additive could be used for mouse models that study the disease.

On top of this, she found that carrageenan causes intestinal and systemic inflammation in animal studies. Considering that inflammation is a well-established factor in most chronic diseases, including heart disease, diabetes, cancer, arthritis, pain disorders, and many others, as a food additive in common use, carrageenan raises serious concerns. Dr. Tobacman also indicates that the amount of carrageenan found in the average American's diet is sufficient to cause inflammation.

Carrageenan is found in common foods, including vegan cheese products, infant formula, ice cream, cream, butter, soy milk, almond milk, rice milk, cottage cheese, sour cream, yogurt, coffee creamers, egg nog, protein supplements, aloe vera gel, deli meats, juices, puddings, pizzas, chocolate bars, coffee beverages, and many other packaged foods. Additionally, some supplements, particularly those involving gel caps, commonly contain carrageenan. And most grocery store rotisserie chickens typically contain the additive.

What Exactly Is Xanthan Gum, and Should You Eat It?

If you've read the labels on packaged vegan cheeses, chances are you've seen xanthan gum listed among the ingredients. Some plant-based cheese cookbooks even include recipes using this odd ingredient. And, like most conscientious people, you probably hesitated, wondering, "What exactly is xanthan gum?" and then reconsidered whether you should purchase the food product. To help you make your own decision, let me share some information about xanthan gum, how it is made, and research on whether this substance is healthy.

Xanthan gum is a carbohydrate secreted by bacteria known as *Xanthomonas campestris*. It is used as a thickener and stabilizing ingredient in packaged foods, including many vegan cheeses and baked goods, particularly gluten-free ones. It is also used in many sauces and condiments, including, for example, McDonald's rib sauce, as well as in toothpastes and medications, including some sustained-release pills. *Xanthomonas campestris* cause a range of plant diseases, so naturally food manufacturers thought, "Let's put these plant-disease-causing bacteria to work for us," or something like that — because everywhere I turn I see xanthan gum in our food supply.

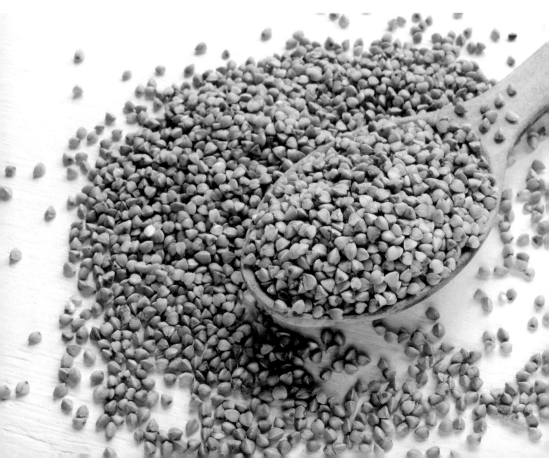

Xanthan gum occurs when *Xanthomonas campestris* bacteria are mixed with fermented sugars, such as corn sugar or sugar from sugar beets, lactose, wheat, or soy, to form a gummy substance. Once the bacteria interact with the fermented sugars, the resulting compound is dried and powdered to form xanthan gum. And yes, the corn, sugar beets, dairy, wheat, and soy used in the production of xanthan gum are likely from genetically modified crops. So if you have allergies to any of these items, when you eat a food item containing xanthan gum, you may be getting more than you bargained for. Further, because wheat may be used in making xanthan gum and wheat also contains gluten, people with celiac disease (an autoimmune disease in which the body adversely reacts to gluten) or those on a gluten-free diet should try to avoid products that use xanthan gum.

Yet xanthan gum is added to many vegan cheese alternatives and gluten-free baked goods because the gum adds elasticity that is otherwise missing in plant-based cheeses and gluten-free grains and flours. In standard baking gluten provides elasticity and texture for breads and baked goods, preventing these items from crumbling; xanthan gum gives gluten-free products a similar elasticity. And in plant-based cheese products, xanthan gum acts as a stand-in for casein, a protein in dairy-based cheeses that helps bind the cheese together and gives it that somewhat rubbery texture we associate with cheese.

While many health experts claim that the mostly indigestible xanthan gum is a harmless food additive, a quick Google search uncovers scores of people posting about their personal difficulties after eating this food ingredient; some people report severe bloating, cramping, and soft stools from xanthan gum–containing foods. And as a nutritionist for many years, I have had many clients ask me whether it's safe to consume. I tell them that I recommend avoiding it as much as possible. Sadly, it has become quite ubiquitous in gluten-free foods, but there is sufficient research to suggest that it harms the gut and causes uncomfortable symptoms like bloating and gas. I suspect further research will demonstrate that it is linked to gut inflammation, which is a precursor to most chronic health conditions.

A couple of years ago the *New York Times* published a story about an infant who died after a xanthan gum–based thickener was added to his formula.[2] He suffered severe bloating and died of necrotizing colitis (NEC), a life-threatening condition in which the bowels are severely damaged. Although there was insufficient evidence to indicate that the xanthan gum thickener had caused the baby's illness and death, the Food and Drug Administration issued a cautionary statement that SimplyThick, a type of xanthan-based product, should not be used in formula for premature infants.[3] Later a study published in the *Journal of Pediatrics* found that xanthan gum may be linked to a delayed onset of NEC in premature infants.[4] But even as the FDA issued the statement advising against the use of the xanthan gum–based thickener with premature infants, it nonetheless recognizes xanthan gum as "generally recognized as safe" (GRAS), even though the government body has not assessed its safety.

In one animal study published in the *Proceedings of the Society for Experimental Biology and Medicine*, researchers found that a diet containing 4 percent xanthan gum caused a 400 percent increase in the amount of water in the intestines as well as an increase in intestinal cell size.[5] Additionally, the same study found that xanthan gum slowed the intestines' absorption of substances; this is cause for concern because most nutrients are absorbed into the blood stream through the lining of the intestinal walls. The study also found that xanthan gum increased the number of sugars present in the intestines, which can cause microbial imbalances in the gut.

But because the FDA states that xanthan gum is generally recognized as safe, few human trials have been conducted. I did find one older human study published in 1993 in the *British Journal of Nutrition* that found that xanthan gum acted as a laxative but also increased flatulence in otherwise healthy men.[6]

So should you eat foods containing xanthan gum? That's entirely up to you, but until there's more scientific evidence supporting its widespread safety claims and we can be sure it is made without GMOs, I'll be keeping xanthan gum off the menu.

Getting Started in Plant-Based Cheese Making

Before we begin our journey into plant-based cheese making, I would first like to introduce you to two more traditional types of cheeses — still using vegan ingredients: yogurt cheese and a traditional almond cheese that is produced using the conventional technique of separating the curds from the whey. While almond milk is a less-than-traditional ingredient, by making this almond cheese you'll learn the process used by conventional cheesemakers. Let's get started.

How to Add Starter Cultures to Make Plant-Based Cheeses

The notion of adding cultures to cheeses may sound technical and difficult or perhaps even a bit scary, but it's none of these. Most commercial dairy-based cheeses are inoculated with a single strain of mold or yeast to give them their signature flavors and cultures. But these monoculture cheeses rarely promote health and nutrition as my plant-based cheeses do. That's because the plant-based cheeses presented here use naturally fermented starter cultures that contain a wider variety and greater numbers of health-building probiotic microbes. Here are some of the starter cultures you can use when making plant-based cheeses:

Miso is a fermented food, typically made from soybeans, although I've seen chickpea and brown rice miso as well. While it is more classically known for its role in miso soup, it also makes a delicious starter culture for plant-based cheeses. You'll find a recipe for one of my favorite aged cheeses, Aged Miso Cheese, that uses miso as a starter culture on page 76.

Probiotic powder: You can find probiotic powder or capsules in the refrigerator section of most health food stores. They usually contain two or more probiotic cultures, some of which include *Lactobacillus acidophilus*, *L. paracasei*, *L. plantarum*, *L. rhamnosus*, *L. salivarius*, *L. delbrueckii subspecies Bulgaricus*, *Bifidobacterium bifidus*, *B. infantis*, *B. lactis*, *B. longum*, or *Streptococcus salivarius subspecies thermophilus*, among others. I find any combination of these probiotics works fine for cheese making as long as the product actually contains live cultures. The test of a probiotic supplement's viability is to make a traditional batch of yogurt to see if it separates the milk — or, in this case, plant-based milk — into curds and whey, which you learned about in the last chapter. I don't recommend probiotic products that use yeast, even beneficial ones, as I find that they tend to create a less-desirable flavored cheese; *Saccharomyces boulardii* is the most common yeast found in probiotic supplements.

Rejuvelac is a fermented grain beverage first created as a health tonic by Ann Wigmore, an early advocate for eating a largely raw-foods, vegetarian diet. Wild microbes feed on the grains soaked in water. If you use rejuvelac as the starter culture for your cheese, simply reduce the amount of liquid called for in the recipe by the amount of rejuvelac you use (so if you use one-half cup of rejuvelac, reduce the amount of water in the recipe by one-half cup), and you'll also be able to eliminate the starter culture called for in the recipe — that is, if you use rejuvelac, you don't have to add probiotic powder or capsules. That will save you money while you still get the health benefits of probiotics. Don't worry if you're not familiar with rejuvelac; I share a recipe for making Gluten-Free, Dairy-Free Rejuvelac on page 60.

Sauerkraut brine: Sauerkraut is made in a saltwater mixture known as brine. Cabbage, apples, and many other fruits and vegetables, which I'll discuss further later in this book, often have a whitish coating on them. Before eating an apple, many people wash or rub off this white coating, but the coating is actually a bloom, which is a mixture of wild microbes that act as starter cultures when making a sauerkraut. Sauerkraut is also made from wild microbes naturally present in the air. The saltwater solution then helps to encourage the growth of beneficial microbes while discouraging harmful ones. When you make your own fermented sauerkraut (and I will show you how in chapter 4), keep the leftover brine full of probiotics and use it as the starter culture for your plant-based cheeses. To do this, as with rejuvelac, simply reduce the amount of liquid in the recipe by the amount of brine you use (so if you use one-half cup of brine, reduce the amount of water called for in the recipe by one-half cup), and you'll also be able to eliminate the starter culture and some of the salt called for in the recipe. That is, if you use brine, you don't have to add probiotic powder or capsules. Once again, this will save you money while you still get all the health benefits of probiotics. Of course, if the recipe calls for sauerkraut brine, then simply follow the directions without making any substitutions.

Whey is the clearish, yellowish liquid that separates from the yogurt or curds when making yogurt or cheese either by using traditional methods of fermenting or by adding an acidifying agent. When we make cheese by heating the milk and then adding an acidifying agent, the resulting whey has no starter cultures and is therefore not valuable in cheese making, so there is no need to save the whey from those cheeses to make fermented cheese recipes. (The recipe for Almond Farmer's Cheese on page 64 is an example of this technique.) You can, of course, save it to add to smoothies or other foods if you'd like, but keep in mind that it doesn't contain any probiotics after it has been heated to the temperature required for cheese making. However, whey that results from making yogurt in the traditional way (such as the recipe for Traditional Vegan Yogurt on page 37) is packed with beneficial lactobacillus bacteria that can give your health a boost and be used in these cheese recipes. If you use whey as the starter for the recipes, simply reduce the amount of liquid called for in the recipe by the amount of whey you use (so if you use one-half cup of whey, reduce the amount of water in the recipe by one-half cup), and you'll also be able to eliminate the starter culture called for in the recipe — that is, if you use whey, you don't have to add probiotic powder or capsules. This will save you money while you still get the health benefits of probiotics.

Yogurt is made with starter cultures from probiotic supplements or from a previous batch of yogurt, a process sometimes called *backslopping*. Depending on the probiotic starter cultures used to make yogurt, it can contain a range of beneficial cultures that are valuable in culturing plant-based cheeses. If you use yogurt as the starter culture for the recipes that follow, simply reduce the amount of liquid called for in the recipe by the amount of yogurt you use (so if you use one-half cup of yogurt, reduce the amount of water in the recipe by one-half cup), and you'll also be able to eliminate the starter culture called for in the recipe. In other words, if you use yogurt, you don't have to add probiotic powder or capsules. This will also save you money while you still get the health benefits of probiotics. Of course, if the recipe already calls for yogurt, then just follow the directions without making any substitutions.

Of course, you can experiment with other microbial-diverse starters for your cheeses, but I encourage you to try these first. You'll find recipes for using each of these items throughout this chapter.

There are many other books and blogs that use some of the starter cultures above, and some of those recipes may ensure the integrity of the probiotics in the final cheese product, but sadly, most don't. When the food containing the probiotic cultures is heated, which many cheese-making recipes call for, the probiotics are destroyed. The resulting cheese may taste good (or not, depending on the recipe), but it won't have any of the health benefits of live cultures because they will be dead.

With the exception of the Almond Farmer's Cheese, which I have included as an example of traditional dairy-style cheese-making techniques, all of the cheese recipes in this book contain live cultures in the final product. You can rest assured that while you're enjoying their rich and delicious flavors you'll also be giving your health a boost with the live cultures found in the cheeses.

The Importance of Filtered Water

It is best to use filtered water when making any recipe for fermented foods because the chlorine found in most tap water kills bacteria, including beneficial ones that are used as starter cultures in making yogurt, cheeses, sauerkraut, kimchi, and other fermented foods. Even water filtered through a water filtration pitcher (be sure to choose one that removes chlorine) is sufficient to significantly improve the outcome of your recipes and ensure they turn out properly.

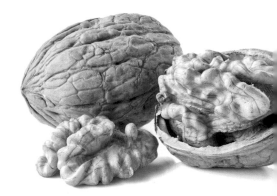

Gluten-Free, Dairy-Free Rejuvelac

A naturally fermented grain beverage first created as a health tonic, rejuvelac doubles as a wild starter culture for plant-based cheese making. Wild microbes naturally present in the air feed on the grains soaked in water, producing probiotic cultures that build health. Remember that if you use rejuvelac as the starter culture for the recipes in this chapter, you should reduce the amount of liquid called for in the recipe by the amount of rejuvelac you use (so if you use one-half cup of rejuvelac, reduce the amount of water in the recipe by one-half cup), and you'll also be able to eliminate the starter culture called for in the recipe — that is, if you use rejuvelac, you don't have to add probiotic powder or capsules. This will save you money while you still get the health benefits of probiotics. For gluten-free rejuvelac you'll want to use gluten-free whole grains such as buckwheat (no relation to wheat), brown rice, millet, quinoa, or oats (be sure to use certified gluten-free ones since oats are often contaminated with gluten-containing grains).

Makes 3 cups

½ cup whole buckwheat grains (or other whole grains of your choice)
3 cups filtered water

Place the grains in a 1-quart glass jar, and add just enough water to cover. Place a double layer of cheesecloth over the mouth of the jar, and secure it in place with a rubber band. Allow the grains to soak for eight hours or overnight; drain, discarding the liquid.

Add 3 cups of filtered water, cover with a fresh cheesecloth, and secure it with a rubber band. Put the jar in a warm place but out of direct sunlight for one to three days. The water will turn whitish-colored and cloudy and will develop a slightly tart flavor. Strain off the grains; these can be reused to make a second batch of rejuvelac if you like. Cover the liquid with a lid, and store in the fridge for up to two weeks.

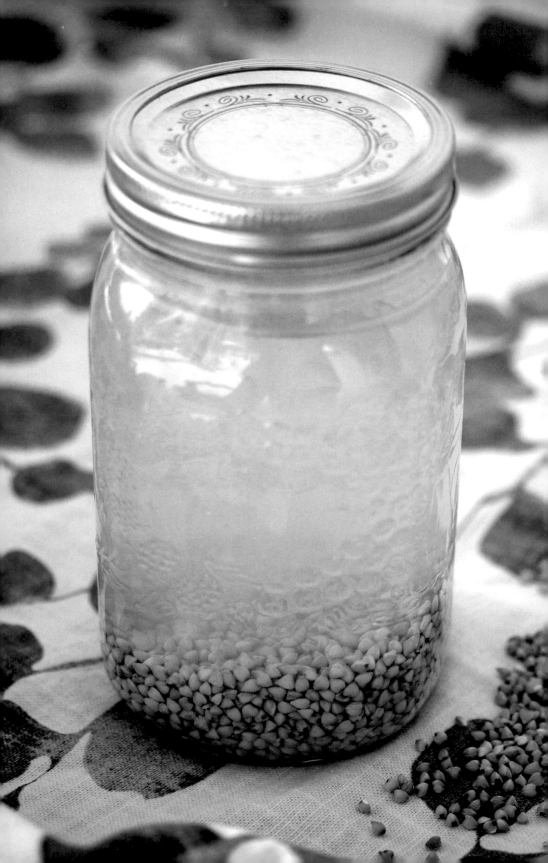

World's Easiest Yogurt Cheese

Yogurt cheese is exactly what it sounds like — cheese made from yogurt. However, most commercial varieties of yogurt are filled with natural or unnatural thickeners like xanthan gum, carrageenan, guar gum, or some other type of thickening agent that interferes with the extraction of excess water from the yogurt to turn it into cheese. As discussed earlier (page 51), for health reasons xanthan gum and carrageenan should be avoided. For best results with this cheese, first make a batch of quality yogurt full of live cultures and devoid of unnatural thickening agents. Because this cheese is made with yogurt that has been made by culturing cashews, it is also full of beneficial microbes. And, as you learned in the last chapter, many commercial varieties of yogurt don't contain any live cultures at all. In other words, by using the cultured cashews, you are guaranteed to get the health-building probiotics you want in your yogurt and yogurt cheese.

Makes about 1 quart/liter

3 cups raw, unsalted cashews
2 cups filtered water
1 probiotic capsule or ¼ teaspoon probiotic powder

In a medium glass or ceramic bowl with a lid, combine the cashews and water, and add the contents of the probiotic capsule, discarding the empty capsule shell, or the probiotic powder; stir together until combined. Cover and let sit for eight to twenty-four hours, depending on how tangy you like your yogurt cheese.

Puree the ingredients in a blender until smooth. Place a cheesecloth-lined sieve over a deep bowl to allow the excess water to drip out of the yogurt. Pour the yogurt into the cheesecloth-lined sieve, and allow it to sit for a few hours until it reaches your desired thickness. You may need to gently squeeze out the excess moisture to ensure the yogurt thickens sufficiently.

Place the yogurt cheese into a cheesecloth-lined mold of your choice, and refrigerate for four to six hours or until firm. You can pull the edges of

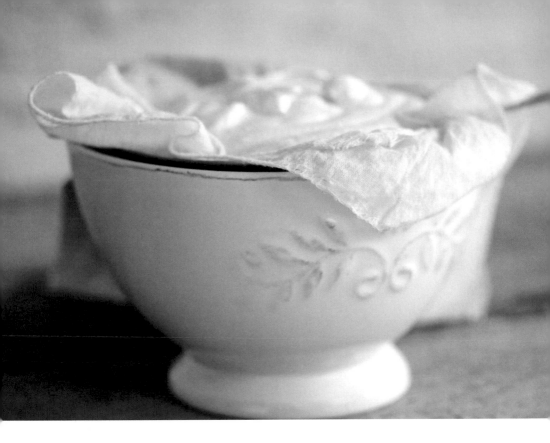

the cheesecloth over the top if you prefer, but it isn't necessary. Remove the cheese from the mold, then peel away the cheesecloth. Serve. Keeps in the refrigerator in a covered container for up to one week.

Choosing Cheese Molds

You can use just about any type of preferred container you want to use as a cheese mold, thereby giving your cheeses a wide range of shapes and sizes. There are professional cheese molds available, but there is no need to use them with these types of cheeses, as most have small holes in them that simply don't work well with the cheeses in this book. Simple Pyrex, glass, or ceramic bowls will work fine. To help you choose the correct size of mold to use, here's what I typically use: a two-cup (472 mL) Pyrex bowl for small blocks of cheese, and a one-quart (952 mL) for medium to large blocks of cheese. But don't feel confined to use only round molds. If you have square or rectangular containers that hold about the same amount, then feel free to use them.

Almond Farmer's Cheese

I call this "farmer's cheese" because it is made using the same type of process as traditional dairy-based farmer's cheese, except that I use almond milk instead of cow's milk. I heat the milk and add an acidifying agent (in this case I've used vinegar), which separates the curds from the whey, and then I further strain it to form a block of cheese. This cheese can be air-dried or not, depending on your preference. You can add herbs or other flavor additions to suit your palate. I love minced fresh basil or thyme in my cheese, but you can select any herbs you prefer. But even without aging or herbs, this cheese is simple and delightful. You can spread it on toast; eat it with fruit, crackers, nuts, or vegetable crudités; serve it with olives or antipasto; or enjoy it with a little fruit jam or coulis (a fruit sauce) as a dessert.

This cheese and other cheeses made in this manner usually don't have any probiotics unless they are added after the milk has cooled and the cheese has been set. Typically, most aged cheeses are inoculated with yeasts or molds at that point — but not always ones that are health promoting. You can age this cheese if you'd like to, although traditionally farmer's cheeses or soft cheeses like this are not aged (i.e., not fermented) and do not contain any probiotics. To age this cheese, follow the instructions outlined in the sidebar "Aging Your Cheeses to Perfection" (see page 71) after you've completed the recipe here.

Makes 1 small block (approximately 2 inches by 3 inches if using a rectangular mold)

1 quart/liter unsweetened almond milk (original flavor, no flavoring added)
1 tablespoon store-bought or homemade apple cider vinegar (see page 134,
     or try using my Crabapple Vinegar on page 129 if you prefer)
Fresh herbs, minced (optional)
1 teaspoon unrefined sea salt

In a medium pot, heat the milk over low heat, stirring occasionally to prevent scalding or sticking. When it looks like the almond milk is just about to boil, remove from the heat; if you prefer to use a candy or canning thermometer (it's not necessary), remove the pot from the stove when the milk reaches 180 to 190°F.

Add the vinegar, stir gently for a few seconds, and then leave it undisturbed for a few minutes. The curds (the solid parts) and whey (the clearish, yellowish fluid) will begin to form and separate.

While the vinegar is working, line a colander with cheesecloth. Once the curds and whey have separated, pour them through it over a sink if you want to discard the whey or over a large bowl if you prefer to keep the whey for later use.

Fold the excess cheesecloth over the curds, and place a clean weight on top; allow it to sit for one to two hours to press out any remaining whey. Alternatively, simply tie up the corners of the cheesecloth, and allow the curds to sit for one to two hours to continue draining.

If using herbs, add them to the cheese after straining and prior to setting up the cheese in a mold (see next step). Alternatively, you can line the bottom of the mold with your desired herbs.

Stir in the salt until it is well combined with the cheese, and place the cheese in a mold or small glass or ceramic bowl and allow to set in the fridge for four to six hours. Serve immediately or store in a covered dish in the refrigerator for up to one week.

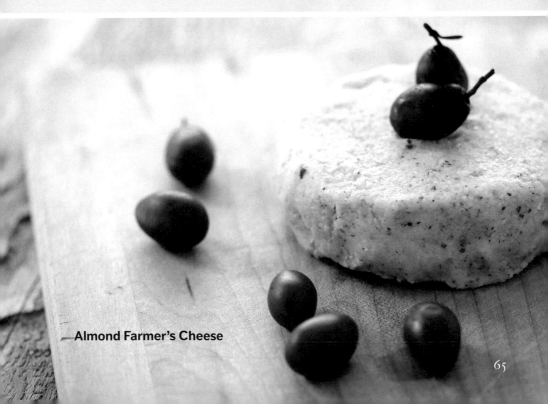

Almond Farmer's Cheese

Walnut Thyme Cheese

This dairy-free cheese has a deliciously salty and savory taste with a rich, buttery texture from the walnuts. The walnuts also give it a distinct but ever-so-mild flavor that makes it unlike any other cheese. Even if you're not a fan of walnuts, I encourage you to buy some high-quality raw walnuts from the refrigerated section in your local health food store. I never liked walnuts (or so I thought) until I tried these fresh ones. I then discovered that I love fresh walnuts — just not the bitter, rancid ones found on most grocery store shelves and in baked goods. Walnuts also offer high amounts of omega 3 fatty acids, which your body needs to protect your brain, maintain a healthy immune system, balance moods, and lessen pain and inflammation in your body. Walnuts are also a good source of vitamins B_6 and E as well as minerals like magnesium and potassium.

This recipe takes only about ten minutes of actual preparation time, but the flavors are superb when the walnuts are allowed to culture for a day. Of course, you can culture it for less time if you simply can't wait to enjoy your next batch. It is delicious on its own, or you can cut it into disks and serve it with your favorite crackers, grapes, or figs. Alternatively, spread it on freshly toasted bread, and savor the rich flavor as it slowly melts from the warmth. Mmmm.

Makes 1 small block

1 cup raw, unsalted walnuts
¼ cup filtered water
2 capsules probiotics or ½ teaspoon probiotic powder
1 teaspoon extra-virgin olive oil
Three 2-inch sprigs fresh thyme, plus a few more for garnish (optional)
1 teaspoon unrefined sea salt
½ cup coconut oil

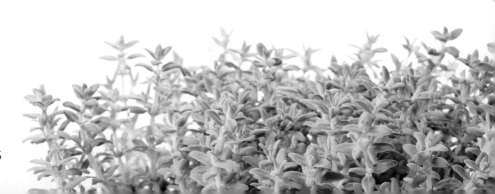

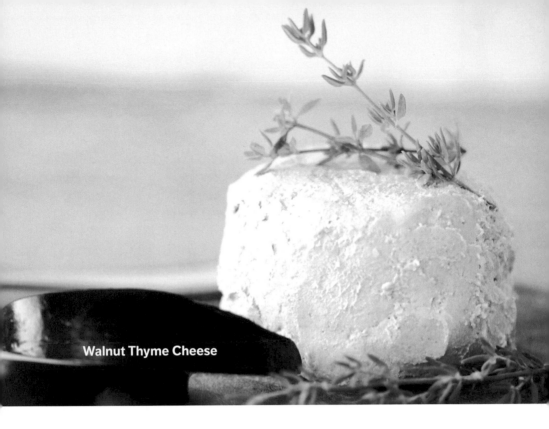

Walnut Thyme Cheese

In a small glass or ceramic bowl, combine the walnuts and water. Empty the contents of the probiotic capsules (discarding the empty capsule shells) or the probiotic powder into the bowl, and stir to combine. Cover and let sit in a warm, undisturbed spot for two days.

In a small frying pan over low to medium heat, sauté the olive oil and thyme until the sprigs are lightly crisped (about 3 to 5 minutes). Remove from the heat. Once cool, pull the thyme leaves off the sprigs, and sprinkle them across the base of a small glass dish.

Pour the walnut mixture into a blender, add the salt and coconut oil, and blend until it is completely smooth; pour it into the glass dish coated in thyme leaves. Refrigerate, uncovered, until it is set (about four hours). Gently remove the cheese from the glass bowl, and serve upside down so the thyme leaves are on the top of the cheese. Garnish with thyme sprigs if desired. It keeps in the refrigerator, covered, for about one month.

Bracotta Cheese

This delightful, slightly sweet, slightly savory cheese has the rich and distinct flavor of Brazil nuts along with a somewhat crumbly texture. I love to crumble it over a mixed green salad with pomegranate arils (seeds) or sliced green apple. It also tastes wonderful simply spread over green and red apple slices or on crackers. Brazil nuts are an excellent source of the mineral zinc, which is imperative to a strong immune system and a healthy prostate, and even helps to fight cancer. Getting your daily requirement of zinc never tasted so good.

Makes about 3 cups or 1 medium-size block

1 cup raw, unsalted Brazil nuts
1 cup raw, unsalted cashews
1 cup filtered water
2 probiotic capsules or ½ teaspoon probiotic powder
⅓ cup coconut oil
1 teaspoon unrefined sea salt
1 tablespoon filtered water

In a small to medium bowl with a lid, combine the Brazil nuts, cashews, and the cup of water. Empty the contents of the probiotic supplements (discarding the empty capsule shells) or probiotic powder into the bowl, and mix together. Allow the mixture to culture for twenty-four to forty-eight hours; the longer fermentation time will develop a stronger flavor for the cheese.

Pour the Brazil nut–cashew mixture into a blender. Add the oil, salt, and 1 tablespoon water, and blend until smooth; this may require effort and a longer blending time to ensure a consistently smooth texture. Pour the mixture into a cheesecloth-lined mold of your choice. Cover and refrigerate until it is set (at least two to four hours).

Remove the cheese from the mold, and unwrap from the cheesecloth. Serve. Refrigerate in a covered container for up to three weeks.

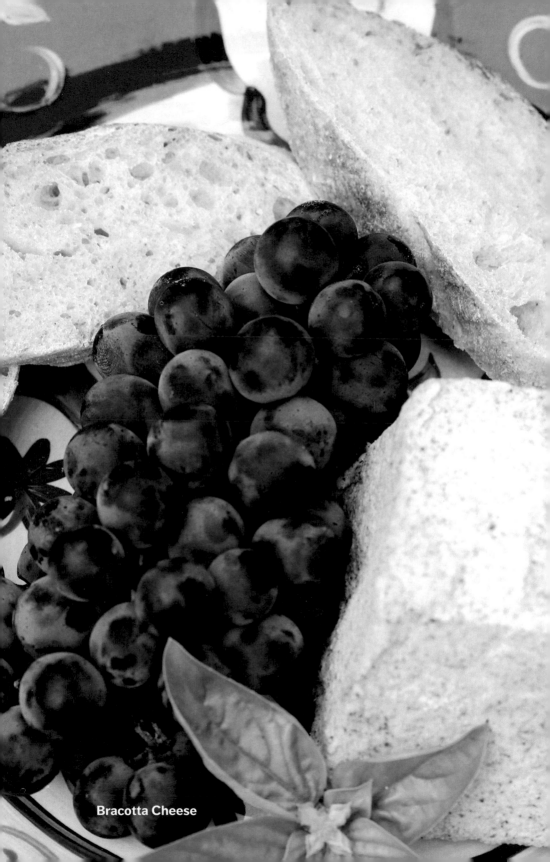

Bracotta Cheese

Chèvrew

This creamy, savory cheese is perfect as an accompaniment to fruit or crackers or on a cheese-and-antipasto platter, but it's also so good that you'll likely eat it on its own now and then. I love it atop a mixed green salad with sweet fruits, particularly peaches or figs, and a handful of pine nuts or pumpkin seeds. You can also serve this cheese with my delicious Cultured Spicy Peach Chutney (page 127). This delightful cheese has a soft texture reminiscent of the goat cheese known as chèvre. This nondairy alternative is one of my favorites and is packed with health-building probiotics. It's so good that you'll probably want to eat it every day — as I do.

Makes about 1½ cups or 1 small block

1 cup raw, unsalted cashews
½ cup filtered water
1 capsule probiotics or ¼ teaspoon probiotic powder
⅓ cup coconut oil
1½ teaspoons unrefined sea salt
Chopped basil for garnish (optional)

In a glass or ceramic bowl, soak the cashews in the water for eight hours or overnight. Blend the cashews and water together until the mixture is smooth and creamy. Pour it into a small glass dish with a lid, empty the capsule of probiotics (discarding the empty capsule shell) or probiotic powder into the cashew mixture, and stir together. Cover with the lid for the dish (if you don't have a dish with a lid, you can use a dish and cover with a clean cloth), and allow the mixture to ferment for twenty-four hours.

Pour the mixture into a blender or food processor, add the oil and salt, and blend together until smooth. Pour it into a small round glass dish lined with cheesecloth. Allow it to chill in the refrigerator until it is firm, or about two to three hours. Garnish with chopped basil if desired, and serve immediately; or store in the refrigerator in a sealed container for up to two weeks.

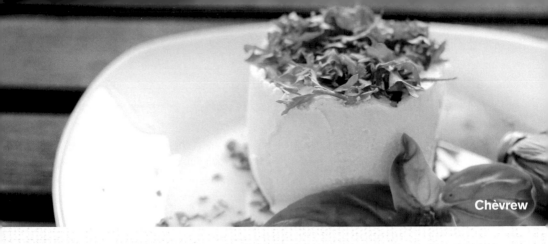
Chèvrew

Aging Your Cheeses to Perfection

There are multiple ways to build the sharper, unique flavors and harder textures that come from aging cheeses. Here are two of my preferred methods:

During the initial soaking and culturing process: When you're soaking nuts or seeds and letting them culture with culturing agents like miso, probiotic powder, rejuvelac, or sauerkraut brine, you can let them culture a little longer than the recipe calls for. Doing so will encourage the proliferation of the natural probiotic bacteria and yeasts found in these agents. When these bacteria and yeasts proliferate they encourage stronger and more distinctive flavors. Keep in mind that at this stage most nuts and seeds can only be cultured for a day or two; after that they will be prone to spoilage, particularly if they are being cultured in warmer temperatures.

During rind development: Some cheeses have a rind or a denser texture that results from building up a rind. You can build a rind on almost any cheese, with the exception of ones that contain fresh herbs or flavor additions like onion or garlic because these items will make the cheese more vulnerable to spoilage. To build a rind, first follow the processes outlined in the recipes within this chapter. Once the cheese has set in its mold, remove it from the mold and gently rub it with one to two teaspoons of noniodized salt. (Iodized salt prevents the growth of microbes, both harmful and beneficial, so is not recommended.) Then let the cheese sit on a fine-mesh wire baking rack. The one I use has gaps that are less than one inch, making the cheese less likely to sag through the gaps and easier to remove after it has been aged the desired amount. You can age the cheeses for a couple of days to a couple of weeks; it may be possible to age them longer, but doing so will risk the formation of mold or other microbes. Of course, if you are familiar with which molds are safe to eat, then you can proceed to age your cheeses for longer periods. This process is also called air-drying because you'll be exposing your cheeses to air, and the air combined with the salt helps wick away excess moisture. You'll need to store them in a cool location for this purpose; I use a clean space in my basement or a room I don't heat in the winter months, but you can use whatever works best for you.

Macadamia Cream Cheese

If you just have to spread cream cheese on bagels or toast, you'll love this dairy-free, fermented version that has all the flavor and loads of probiotics to give your health a boost. This delicious and creamy dairy-free cream cheese has a delicate macadamia nut flavor. Unlike dairy-based cream cheeses, this cheese is packed with health-promoting beneficial bacteria. It's simple to make but does need about twelve hours to culture and a couple of hours to set.

Makes 1 small block

½ cup raw, unsalted macadamia nuts
½ cup raw, unsalted cashews
½ cup filtered water, plus 3 tablespoons
1 probiotic capsule or ¼ teaspoon probiotic powder
3 fresh Medjool dates, pitted
⅓ cup coconut oil
¼ teaspoon unrefined sea salt

In a glass or ceramic bowl, combine the macadamia nuts, cashews, ½ cup water, and the probiotic capsule (discarding the empty capsule shell) or probiotic powder; stir until mixed, and cover. In a separate bowl mix the dates with the remaining 3 tablespoons of water, and cover. Allow both to sit overnight for twelve hours.

In a blender combine both mixtures, add the salt, and blend until smooth. Add the coconut oil and continue blending. You may need to push the ingredients down with a spatula a few times to ensure a creamy, smooth consistency. Pour into a cheesecloth-lined dish or mold. Refrigerate for one to two hours, or until it is set. Serve. Store in the refrigerator, covered, for up to one month.

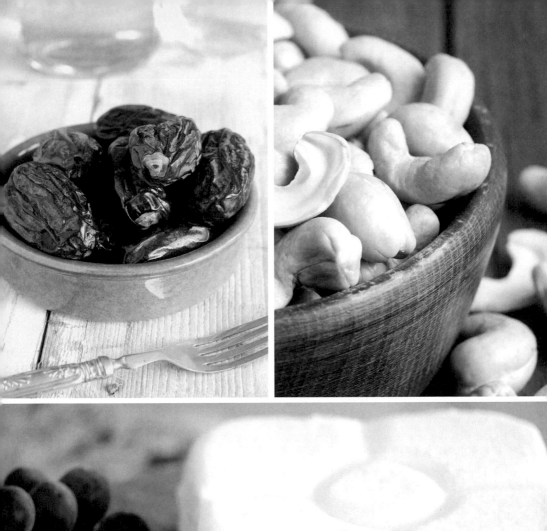

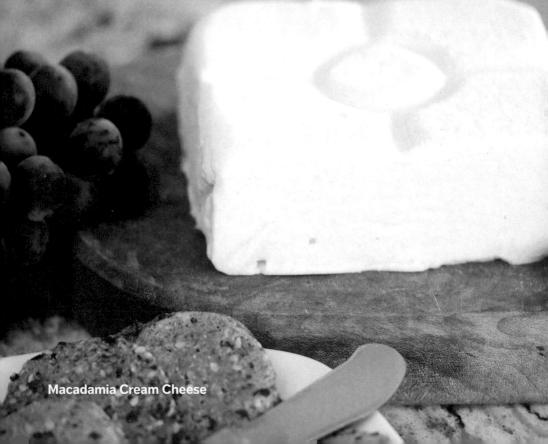

Macadamia Cream Cheese

Aged Smoked Cheese

To me the combination of cheese and a natural smoky flavor and aroma couldn't be better. Because I love both flavors, I developed the following recipe to bring them together with a nondairy option at last. But don't worry: I won't have you standing over a smoker, trying to infuse flavor into your cheese; instead, simply using smoked salt both for inside the cheese as well as to develop a rind saves you time and energy, but you'll still end up with a deliciously smoky block of cheese that you can slice, melt, spread on crackers, or enjoy on its own. Don't worry about "making a rind" — all you really need to do is rub salt over the cheese block and allow it to air-dry in a cool room until it has developed a firm outer coating.

Makes 1 medium-size block

2 cups raw, unsalted cashews
1 cup filtered water
2 probiotic capsules or ½ teaspoon probiotic powder
½ cup coconut oil
4 teaspoons smoked unrefined sea salt, divided

In a glass or ceramic bowl with a lid, combine the cashews and water, and empty the probiotic capsules (discarding the empty capsule shells) or probiotic powder into the cashew-water mixture, and stir until combined. Cover and let sit for twenty-four hours.

Pour the cultured cashews and their liquid into a blender. Add the oil and 2 teaspoons of the salt, and blend until smooth. You may need to push the ingredients down with a spatula a few times to ensure a creamy, smooth consistency.

Pour the cheese mixture into a cheesecloth-lined bowl that is the shape you'd like the finished cheese to be. Refrigerate for four to six hours, or until it is firm. Remove the cheese from the bowl, and peel away the cheesecloth.

Gently rub the remaining 2 teaspoons of salt over the full surface of the cheese, including the bottom. Carefully place the cheese on a wire rack in a cool, dark, and undisturbed place, and allow the cheese to air-dry for seven to twenty-eight days, or longer if desired. After you have aged the cheese, refrigerate and serve, or store in a covered container in the refrigerator for up to one month.

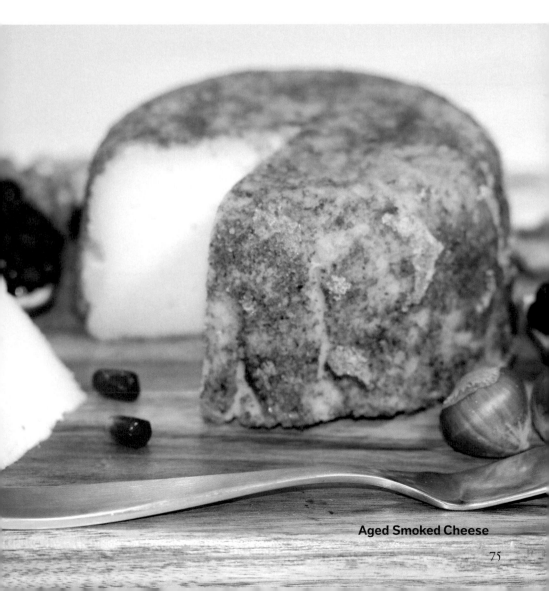

Aged Smoked Cheese

Aged Miso Cheese

Earlier I mentioned that there are many types of starter cultures that can be used in plant-based cheese making. Miso is one of my favorites. Its mild, naturally aged, rich, slightly nutty flavor beautifully lends itself to aged plant-based cheeses.

I recently started a new holiday tradition in which I begin making this cheese at the beginning of December. Once the initial culturing process is done, I form the cheese block, rub it with sea salt, and set it on a wire mesh rack in a cool space to allow it to ferment for the remaining days until Christmas Eve. Then Curtis and I enjoy a beautiful holiday cheese platter with this cheese as the star. With three weeks of aging time, it develops a firm texture and a sharp taste that is delightful with pomegranate arils (seeds), mandarin oranges, walnut halves, and figs, making it the perfect Christmas cheese and a wonderful, unique holiday tradition in our home.

Makes 1 medium-size block

2 cups raw, unsalted cashews
1 cup filtered water
1 tablespoon dark miso
3 teaspoons unrefined sea salt, divided
½ cup coconut oil

In a glass or ceramic bowl with a lid, combine the cashews, water, and miso, and stir until they are combined. Cover and let sit for twenty-four hours.

Pour the cultured cashews into a blender. Add 1 teaspoon of the salt as well as the oil, and blend until smooth. You may need to push the ingredients down with a spatula a few times to ensure a creamy, smooth consistency.

Pour the cheese mixture into a cheesecloth-lined bowl that is the shape you'd like the finished cheese to be. Refrigerate for four to six hours, or until it is firm. Remove the cheese from the bowl, and peel away the cheesecloth.

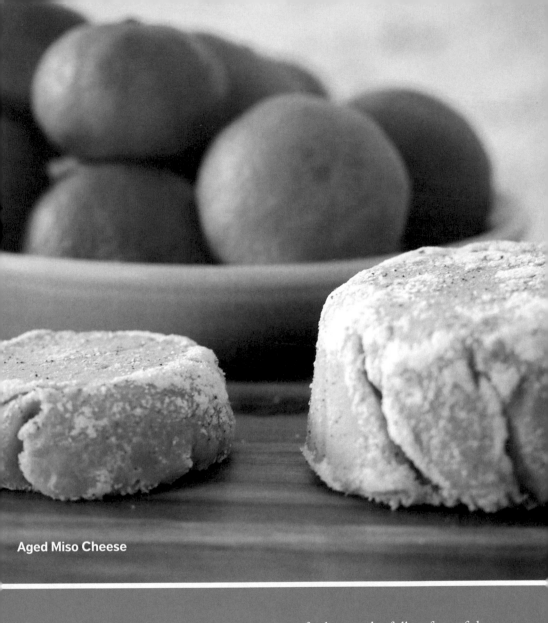

Aged Miso Cheese

Gently rub the remaining 2 teaspoons of salt over the full surface of the cheese, including the bottom. Carefully place it on a wire rack in a cool, dark, and undisturbed place, and allow the cheese to air-dry for seven to twenty-eight days, or longer if desired. After you have aged the cheese, refrigerate and serve, or store in a covered container in the refrigerator for up to one month.

Aged Savorella Cheese

Sauerkraut brine is another one of the starter cultures that can be used in plant-based cheese making. When you make this cheese from homemade sauerkraut, you can be sure it will be full of health-building probiotic cultures that naturally age the cheese. The brine also contains nutrients like sulforaphane, pulled from the cabbage as it ferments. If you make this cheese with store-bought sauerkraut brine, make sure to choose sauerkraut that has not been pasteurized; it should come from the refrigerator section of your health food or grocery store and should say "unpasteurized" or "live cultures" on the label. Using sauerkraut brine as a starter imparts a delicious, naturally aged, sharp, and rich flavor to the cheese.

Makes 1 medium-size block

2 cups raw, unsalted cashews
²⁄₃ cup filtered water
⅓ cup sauerkraut brine
3 teaspoons unrefined sea salt, divided
½ cup coconut oil

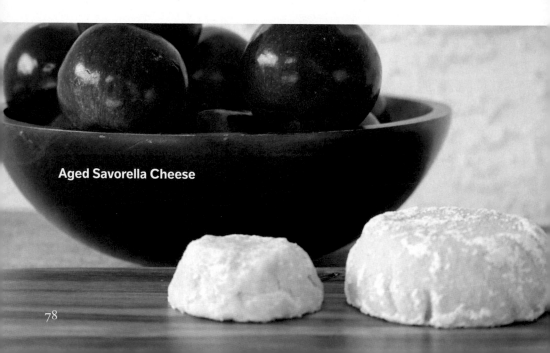

Aged Savorella Cheese

In a glass or ceramic bowl with a lid, combine the cashews, water, and brine, and stir well. Cover and let sit for twenty-four hours.

Pour the cultured cashews and their liquid into a blender. Add 1 teaspoon of the salt as well as the oil, and blend until smooth. You may need to push the ingredients down with a spatula a few times to ensure a creamy, smooth consistency.

Pour the cheese mixture into a cheesecloth-lined bowl that is the shape you'd like the finished cheese to be. Refrigerate for four to six hours, or until it is firm. Remove from the bowl, and peel away the cheesecloth.

Gently rub the remaining 2 teaspoons of salt over the full surface of the cheese, including the bottom. Carefully place it on a wire rack in a cool, dark, and undisturbed place, and allow the cheese to air-dry for two weeks. After you have aged the cheese, refrigerate and serve, or store in a covered container in the refrigerator for up to one month.

Interview with Artisanal Plant-Based Cheesemaker Karen McAthy

When I discovered Blue Heron Creamery cultured vegan cheeses made in Vancouver, British Columbia, Canada, I had to get in touch with the owner and chef behind the plant-based delights. As an avid artisanal cheesemaker myself, I am always happy to learn about the techniques and flavors others are using in order to both develop my cultured cheese-making art as well as share the teachings with my readers. Chef Karen McAthy, the mastermind behind the aged plant-based, dairy-free cheeses, was kind enough to share some of her secrets to great cultured cheese making. She applies many traditional cheese-making techniques to plant-based ingredients. While I use some of these techniques, most of the cheeses I make are made with different methods. But I am happy to share her responses so you can try a variety of techniques if you like.

What are your favorite vegan cheese ingredients?

With respect to ingredients, I enjoy using a variety of nuts, seeds, and legumes. "Favorite" is not really how I think of any one ingredient. I consider each ingredient in relation to how I intend to use it and the results it produces. Cashews are very common in vegan cheese making, and I, of course, use them a lot, but I have really developed an affinity for almonds and their ability to be aged into very sharp, hard cheeses. Hazelnuts, walnuts, and chick-peas are also something I'm starting to use more heavily, and I am having some interesting results. Hazelnuts can withstand longer aging times without becoming rancid or too sour, and this allows for complexity and depth of flavor to develop, so this is of particular interest to me.

How do you get the cheeses to be creamy?

This is all about the culturing process. I don't use fillers such as starches or gums, and I don't add oil to any of my cheeses. Creaminess is about finding the right cultures and the right culturing conditions (time, humidity, etc.). The cultures (bacteria, molds, yeasts) eat the proteins and sugars and convert the base, just as they do in dairy cheese making. Time and practice and taking notes on each effort so I can compare and learn each time I make a batch allow me to track what variables have the most impact on the texture of the cheese.

What are your favorite flavor additions?

I only occasionally add flavors to the cheeses I make....I have been very focused on work-ing with the cultures to understand what flavors result from their activity. However, I do really like including dried fruits such as apricot and figs or herbs such as tarragon. I also like to work with wine and beer for developing flavor through rind washing or adding into thickened/aging curd.

How do you get the cheeses to hold or bind together?

Again, this is about culturing, aging, and the removal of excess moisture. Achieving a high-quality curd is the first most important step. The curd is the by-product of the cul-tures acting on the nut milks, and this is thicker than any "whey" or moisture that separates. Draining this off and allowing the curd to clump together is essential before adding other ingredients or forming into molds.

After molding — or even sometimes during the molding process — I use thick butter muslin or thin, plain (unbleached) canvas to help with wicking away excess moisture. Doing so requires daily monitoring and changing the muslin/canvas in order to avoid unwelcome microbes from growing. Also, during this process I flip and turn the cheeses frequently, allowing moisture to evaporate.

I also use a cheese press for some of the cheeses that I make, and this allows for con-sistently applied pressure to squeeze out moisture while keeping the cheese compressed into the desired shape.

What is your favorite cheese that you've created?

This changes! Right now, though, it is an almond cheese that we call Beachwood. It takes several months to age properly, is quite hard, slices very thinly, shaves a little like a

Parmesan Reggiano, and is sharp and tangy. We inoculate the rind with culture, then wash the rind repeatedly, then smoke the cheese, and finish the process with several washing/drying steps using a kelp stout from Tofino Brewing. This cheese has smokiness and an umami quality that is intense but not overpowering, and this makes it great for using with other culinary applications.

How do you build a rind on your cheeses? I've used salting and air-drying, but I'm curious if you have other techniques you like to use.

Rind formation depends on the type of cheese I am making. I use ashes, or molds/cultures, or beer and wine to wash, and salt, of course. A highly concentrated saline brine is great for washing cheeses and getting them to express excess moisture and form a firm rind on the surface of the cheese. All of these methods require air-drying/aging after application or washing/soaking time. I have tested using dehydrators on low/no heat setting for a more rapid removal of moisture, but this is not my favorite way of achieving a rind.

What forms of microbial starters do you use? I know some people use rejuvelac, while others use specific cultures from their favorite cheese-making suppliers.

I use a number of different microbial starters and secondary cultures. I feed my cultures on plant-based mediums over a few generations to train them, and I am working on a process to replicate and store them in this manner.

Lactic acid starters I use include a number of mesophilic direct set cultures, kefir cultures (trained on coconut milk or nut milk), rejuvelac, plant-based probiotic capsules… yogurt cultures, again from plant-based yogurt making. I've also used kombucha and tempeh cultures.

I use a wide array of secondary cultures for rind blooming, and those may include yeasts such as candida, or camembert. I have been working to create my own combination of these, applied in different stages to find the results I like best.

Karen McAthy
The Art of Plant-Based Cheesemaking: How to Craft Real, Cultured, Non-Dairy Cheeses
Chef, Blue Heron Creamery
Vancouver, BC, Canada

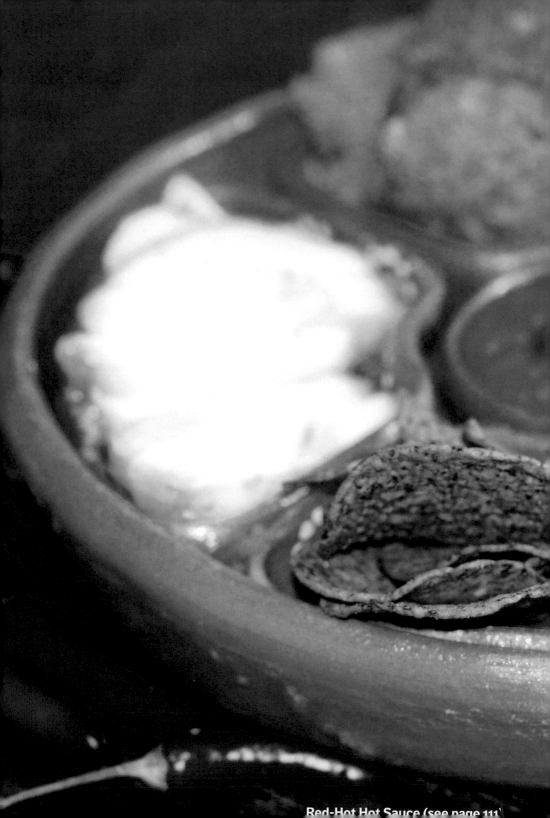

Red-Hot Hot Sauce (see page 111)

CHAPTER FOUR

SAUERKRAUT, PICKLES, AND CULTURED VEGETABLES

My paternal grandmother, Helma Schoffro, was an amazing French Canadian woman who was ahead of her time. Originally named Helma Simoneau, she worked as a French-English translator for the head of Ford Motor Company in the early twentieth century. After meeting my grandfather, Joe Schoffro, they decided to settle in southern Ontario to start a family and farm. My grandfather held down a full-time position as the manager of the largest store in the town of Simcoe — Woolworth's — and spent the rest of his time working on their massive farm that my grandmother built up and managed full time while raising their ten children, one of whom is my father, Michael Schoffro. My dad helped with just about every function on the farm, from tending to the chickens to ploughing, planting, and harvesting the fields.

They cultivated a huge organic fruit and vegetable garden. Whenever I'd visit I'd hang out in the kitchen with my grandmother for a short time before she tasked me with picking whatever vegetables or fruits she needed for the day's meals. I'd pick green beans, cabbage, kohlrabi, raspberries, and many other fruits and vegetables, depending on what was in season and the meals my grandmother was making that day. Having spent so much time picking produce during my childhood, I was usually fairly quick at the task — except during raspberry season, when I ate one or two raspberries for every one that found its way into my basket.

My grandmother made all sorts of foods that she preserved and kept in their huge walk-in cellar beneath their home. I don't recall all the items she made, but there always seemed to be a supply of sauerkraut and dandelion wine among the vast number of food items. Nothing ever went to waste. She found a way to use everything that came up in the garden, and she fed the vegetable scraps to the hens, who would lay eggs for other meals. She was truly living an organic and sustainable life long before it became fashionable. She just knew that this way of living — we now call it homesteading — was in harmony with the earth and supported the health of her family. That was good enough for her.

While I frequently helped make meals, I never learned the art of sauerkraut making from my grandmother, but that didn't stop me from eating a whole lot of this delicious fermented cabbage dish she originally learned from my grandfather, who came as a boy to Canada from Austria. As an adult looking back, I became inspired by her amazing food and cooking skills, so I decided to learn how to make sauerkraut. This was before the dawn of blogging and Pinterest, so I devoured book after book to prepare myself for my newfound interest. Nervous about the proposition, I carefully followed every instruction to the letter. After the fermentation wait time was over, I gingerly removed the lid to the crock, the weights, and plate that covered the cabbage, revealing fresh sauerkraut that tasted better than any of the bottled varieties I had tried. I was instantly hooked and realized that these simple techniques could be applied to almost any vegetable. As my husband, Curtis, can attest, I have fermented almost every different variety of vegetable in one form or another — as sauerkraut, pickles, kimchi, or other fermented vegetable delights.

Before he met me, Curtis had never tasted sauerkraut, so I was happy to share with him from one of my fresh batches. He loved his first taste of my homemade sauerkraut so much that he ate it almost every day that week, so I nicknamed him Krautis to honor his newfound love of sauerkraut.

In this chapter I'll share some of my favorite sauerkraut recipes along with step-by-step instructions to guide you through the process of making your own sauerkraut. I know from experience that it can feel a bit intimidating at first, but once you've made your first batch, you'll discover how easy it is and will want to make a lot more. I'll also share some of the health benefits of sauerkraut, kimchi, curtido, cultured pickles, and other forms of pickled vegetables. Once you've learned the basic brining technique, you can use it to experiment with a wide variety of fermented foods.

Here are the delicious sauerkrauts and pickles you'll learn how to make in this chapter:

- Basic Sauerkraut
- Spiced Sauerkraut
- Five-Minute Broccoli Sauerkraut
- Pineapple Sauerkraut
- Purple Sauerkraut
- Spicy Dill Fermented Pickles
- Salvadoran Salsa
- Star Anise Carrots
- Cultured Onions
- Red-Hot Hot Sauce
- Fermented Chopped Salad
- Dill Cucumber Pickle Bites
- Zucchini Pickles
- Taco Pickles
- White Kimchi

Sauerkraut: The Ancient Superfood with Modern Uses

Even as a child I enjoyed sauerkraut — mostly heaped over hot dogs with a generous amount of mustard. Perhaps that was your first taste of this sour fermented cabbage dish too? I instantly loved its unique sour and tart flavor. As an adult I began experimenting with many sauerkraut combinations.

There is much more to sauerkraut than just a hot dog topping. This unique German staple can be made with many additions that impart flavor nuances to whatever you eat it with — and it tastes great on its own too! I'll discuss more of the flavor options, but first let's explore all the reasons why you'll want to give sauerkraut a more prominent place in your diet.

Ten Reasons to Love Sauerkraut

In addition to its deliciously tart taste, sauerkraut (with live cultures) is getting rave reviews from exciting research that showcases its many health benefits when eaten on a regular basis. Here are some of the best reasons to love the fermented cabbage:

1. Fungus fighter: What if I told you that sauerkraut contains beneficial bacteria that are miniature antifungal manufacturing facilities? It sounds more like science fiction than science fact, but it is true. Research published in the *Journal de Mycologie Medicale* found that some of the probiotics in sauerkraut produce compounds that kill some species of Candida fungi, which frequently cause vaginal or intestinal infections.[1]

2. Athletic performance booster: Let's face it: you probably never think of sauerkraut among the foods or supplements that enhance athletic performance. But perhaps when word gets out about sauerkraut's impressive performance-enhancing properties, it will become the fitness food of choice among athletes everywhere. That's because research published in *Current Sports Medicine Reports* found numerous sports-performance benefits from eating probiotic-rich foods, including reducing allergic conditions and aiding recovery from fatigue as well as improving immune function.[2] If Popeye were still around, he'd probably switch from spinach to sauerkraut to keep his muscles strong and energy levels high.

3. Heart healer: Taste alone is a great reason to enjoy more sauerkraut, but heart health joins the ever-growing list of reasons to eat this fermented superfood. Research published in the medical journal *Food and Function* found that unpasteurized sauerkraut contained a potent probiotic known as wild *Lactobacillus plantarum*, to which many of sauerkraut's heart-healing abilities could be attributed.[3]

The scientists found that the probiotic-rich sauerkraut reduced cholesterol and triglyceride levels and increased levels of two powerful antioxidants, superoxide dismutase (SOD) and glutathione, which eliminate harmful free radicals — charged molecules that damage tissues and cells in the body, including the heart and blood vessels. Additionally, sauerkraut reduced the degradation of fats in the body (a process known as lipid peroxidation), which is linked to heart disease.

4. Breast cancer preventer: Cabbage, along with other foods in the cruciferous family of vegetables, has been long known to have anticancer properties, but when fermented with live cultures, it gets even better. The fermentation process actually converts the anticancer compounds in cabbage, known as glucosinolates, to a more active and functional form called isothiocyanates, well-established cancer fighters. But you don't need to remember their names to know that sauerkraut helps fight cancer. According to scientists at the Department of Food Science and Human Nutrition at the University of Illinois at Urbana-Champaign, regularly eating fermented cabbage can help to regulate estrogen levels.[4] Because high levels of estrogen have been linked with the development of estrogen-dependent breast cancers, this is yet one more way sauerkraut exerts its anticancer influence.

5. Hormone regulator: Because sauerkraut can help reduce excessive levels of estrogen, it may also help treat many other hormonally linked health concerns, including menstrual difficulties and mood imbalances, which are both frequently linked with high levels of estrogen.

6. Food poisoning preventer: Research shows that the beneficial microbes that cultivate during the process of fermenting cabbage kill harmful bacteria. In one study *E. coli* bacteria (the kind that cause food poisoning) were artificially implanted into sauerkraut. Normally, inoculating food with these harmful bacteria would cause the food to become contaminated and cause food poisoning for anyone who ate it. But in this study researchers found that the probiotics *Lactobacillus plantarum* and *L. mesenteroides*, which form naturally

during the fermentation process, actually went to battle with the *E. coli* bacteria and, in just a few days, completely destroyed them until they were no longer present in the sauerkraut. And research shows that probiotics found in sauerkraut demonstrate antibacterial activity against numerous other harmful bacteria linked to food poisoning as well. If sauerkraut can kill harmful bacteria in a ceramic crock, imagine what it can do for your body. Even most antibiotic drugs are completely useless against these potent harmful invaders. But sauerkraut makes light work of these nasty critters.

7. Virus inhibitor: Sauerkraut frequently contains the beneficial bacteria *L. plantarum*, which has been found to have antiviral effects. This makes sauerkraut a potential treatment for colds, flu, chronic fatigue syndrome, and possibly even Ebola or HIV.

8. Gut protector: With so many beneficial bacteria found in sauerkraut, enjoying it on a regular basis is a great way to boost your gastrointestinal (GI) tract health.

9. Nutritional booster: When cabbage and other nutritious ingredients are fermented to become sauerkraut, and the numbers and varieties of beneficial microbes significantly increase, you actually get even more nutrition from these vegetables. The probiotics that accompany the vegetables make the food's nutrients more absorbable to the body.

10. Taste enhancer: Sauerkraut is delicious on its own, on top of your favorite vegan or turkey hot dog, on a black bean burger, or as a side dish to accompany just about any type of meal. It tastes great and is extremely versatile. Check out my list of thirteen ways to eat more sauerkraut on pages 89–90.

Sadly, however, most of the sauerkraut available in grocery stores is not the health food it should be. Many commercial sauerkraut manufacturers have taken shortcuts in making their sauerkrauts in order to increase their profits: instead of waiting for natural fermentation to occur, many instead employ an artificial pickling process using white vinegar, which doesn't contain any probiotics. Even those companies that stay true to natural processes still frequently pasteurize their sauerkraut so it can remain on grocery store shelves for longer periods. This pasteurization, or heating process, during bottling kills any live cultures needed for the health benefits of sauerkraut. So if you're buying sauerkraut, be sure to choose only products with live cultures, found in the refrigerator section of your health food or grocery store. Better yet, make your own at home — as you'll soon discover, it's easier than you think.

Making Your Own Sauerkraut

If you've never made your own sauerkraut but are thinking you would like to start, I'm thrilled to be part of your fermentation journey. As I mentioned earlier, I was excited to make my first batch of kraut (and still get excited with each new batch), anticipating its completion every day while I waited weeks for the fermentation process to convert cabbage into sauerkraut.

You'll be happy to know that you won't need many pieces of special equipment. Even a large mason jar can double as a fermentation crock if you don't have one. However, if you're thinking of making your own sauerkraut on a regular basis, you might want to invest in a crock with a plate that fits inside, food-safe nonmetallic weights, and a wooden spoon or tamper. You'll also need to have on hand unrefined finely ground sea salt (iodized salt won't work because the iodine kills beneficial bacteria), filtered water (preferably unchlorinated water since chlorine also kills probiotics), and of course, cabbage.

Once you've made your first batch of sauerkraut you'll find that doing it again and again is simple. Even if you're not a fan of the traditional-tasting store-bought sauerkraut, creating unique and delicious flavor combinations simply by adding different ingredients is easy: apple-cabbage, garlic and chili, curry-cauliflower, beet and red cabbage, seaweed and ginger — the options are endless. I urge you to give it a try.

While sauerkraut may be the traditional garnish for hot dogs and sausage, there are many other pairings to help you get more sauerkraut into your diet. Here are thirteen ways for you to enjoy sauerkraut:

1. On Reuben sandwiches. While traditionally made from corned beef and pastrami, you can also choose one of the vegan meat options available if you prefer.

2. Atop pizzas and flatbread. Add sauerkraut at the end of the cook time to make sure you preserve sauerkraut's health-boosting probiotics.
3. As a garnish on soup.
4. On pulled pork, pulled chicken, or pulled vegetarian sandwiches. My sister, Bobbi Meyer, makes amazing vegetarian "pulled pork" sandwiches in her café, Sweet Greens, in Hagersville, Ontario, using cooked, grated carrots smothered in a homemade barbecue sauce.
5. Over or with bean dishes.
6. With pierogis.
7. Alongside shepherd's pie or a veggie version.
8. On burgers or veggie burgers.
9. With pretzels.
10. With roasted garlic-and-herb potatoes.
11. Over a bowl of brown rice.
12. Over a bowl of brown-rice or other whole-grain noodles. Then top with grated carrots and green onions for a quick and easy meal.
13. On its own. Who says sauerkraut must be a garnish? Why not serve up a bowl of sauerkraut on its own?

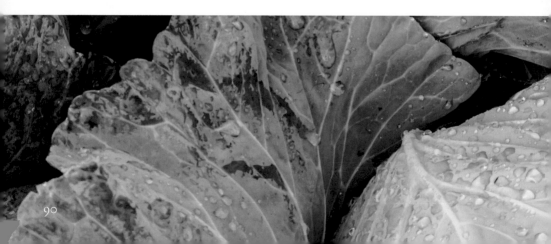

Basic Sauerkraut

When it comes to probiotic-rich foods, yogurt gets all the fanfare, but sauerkraut with live cultures contains a wider variety of probiotic strains and, arguably, more health benefits. But why choose between the two when you can enjoy both foods?

Sadly, the art of making homemade sauerkraut has dwindled over the years. Most people wrongly assume that it takes a lot of work and is difficult to make, but it actually requires minimal effort and is quite simple once you get used to it.

The following recipe is for making a simple sauerkraut without the many possible flavor additions. It is delicious on its own, but feel free to add a handful of flavor additions, such as caraway seeds, fennel seeds, coriander seeds, juniper berries, fresh basil, fresh or dried rosemary, mustard seeds, or others. Use your imagination if you want to try different flavors of sauerkraut, but feel free to also enjoy this simple sauerkraut recipe as is because it has a great flavor all on its own.

The description below may seem intensive, but once you get used to the basic process, it's actually very easy. The technique to make probiotic-rich vegetable dishes usually involves brining, a process in which vegetables are fermented in a saltwater solution — brine is simply the saltwater solution. The salt draws water out of the cabbage and helps protect the vegetables from microorganisms that decompose food. Many probiotic bacteria still grow in the salt solution; however, if you use too much salt, then no microorganisms can survive and fermentation won't take place.

You can use a variety of fermentation vessels, ranging from small to large stoneware crocks, ceramic or glass bowls, or wide-mouthed mason jars. Avoid using metal or plastic containers, as these will cause the level of acidity to increase, which can result in a chemical reaction with the metal or plastic. The probiotics are destroyed by the metal, while the plastic can leech into the food, resulting in unsafe chemical exposure. Many plastics, even ones free from bisphenol A, still contain toxic, hormone-disrupting ingredients that are best avoided. Additionally, most beneficial microbes do not grow well in a metal container, so they are best avoided. Glass, ceramic, or stoneware are best.

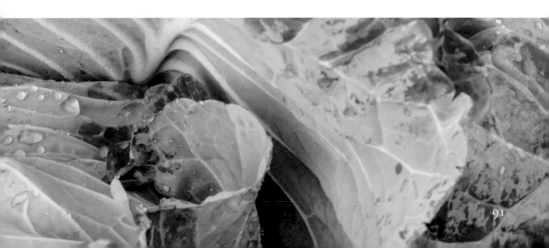

Whatever type you use, you'll need a plate, jar, or cover that fits *inside* the crock, bowl, or jar to help submerge the vegetables that would otherwise float to the top and potentially spoil. For the cover I use a plate as large as I can find. Flea markets and antique shops are great places to find both crocks and plates of different sizes to fit together. Then, you'll need a weight that will be placed on top of the plate to keep the vegetables submerged. I sometimes use a bowl filled with extra salt water, but you can also use a rock that has been scrubbed and boiled for at least fifteen minutes. A one-gallon glass jug tends to be a great weight for larger crocks, and mason jars filled with water make good weights for smaller crocks or bowls.

Don't panic if you open your crock after a couple of weeks to find a disgusting mold growing on top. It can be scooped off the surface, and as long as the mold has not penetrated deeper within the crock, you will still have a perfectly good sauerkraut.

Makes approximately 3 to 4 quarts

2 small to medium heads green cabbage, shredded
1 tablespoon juniper berries, coarsely cracked with a mortar and pestle or pepper mill (optional)
3 tablespoons unrefined fine sea salt or 6 tablespoons unrefined coarse sea salt
1 quart (or liter) filtered water

Place the green cabbage in a large, clean crock or a large glass or ceramic bowl; push it down with your clean fist or a wooden spoon to release the juices. Add a pinch of the juniper berries throughout the process of adding cabbage.

In a pitcher or a large measuring cup, dissolve the salt in the water, stirring if necessary to encourage the salt to dissolve. Pour the saltwater over the cabbage until it is submerged, leaving a couple of inches of room at the top for the cabbage to expand.

Place a plate that fits inside the crock or bowl over the cabbage-water mixture, and weigh it down with food-safe weights or a bowl or jar of water, making sure the vegetables remain submerged under the brine as they ferment. (Ideally, choose the biggest plate possible to fit inside the crock and provide the greatest amount of surface coverage to prevent cabbage pieces from floating to the top of the crock.) Cover with a lid or a cloth, and allow it to ferment for at least two weeks, checking periodically to ensure that the cabbage mixture is still submerged below the water line. After two weeks the sauerkraut will still be fairly crunchy; if you like a more traditional sauerkraut, allow it to ferment longer to soften the cabbage further.

If any mold forms on the surface of the crock, simply scoop it out. It will not spoil the sauerkraut unless it gets deeper inside the crock. It may form where the mixture meets the air, but it rarely forms deeper inside the crock.

After two weeks, or longer if you prefer, dish out the sauerkraut into jars or a bowl, cover, and place in the fridge, where it will last for at least a few months to a year.

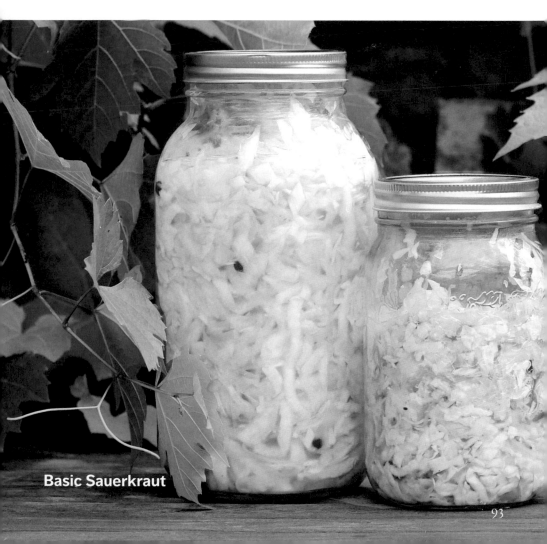

Basic Sauerkraut

Spiced Sauerkraut

If you love the taste of spicy pickles, you'll love this sauerkraut. It has a mild "kick" that you can easily increase simply by adding more cayenne chili peppers. You can also substitute milder chilis like jalapeños if you prefer a little less heat. Whenever I want spicy food I open my crock full of spicy sauerkraut. Once you've made a crock of this sauerkraut, you'll have a delicious dish you can enjoy for months. Serve it on its own or over brown or black rice for a quick and easy meal. It's also the perfect condiment for everything from your favorite sausage to a salad or wrap when you want to add some heat and flavor. The garlic offers heart-healing benefits, the chilis help reduce pain and inflammation throughout the body, and, as stated earlier, the fermented cabbage has potent anticancer compounds.

Makes approximately 2 quarts

1 large or 2 small heads green cabbage, shredded
6 dried or fresh whole cayenne chilis (or more for a hotter sauerkraut)
3 garlic cloves, minced
4 tablespoons unrefined fine sea salt or 8 tablespoons unrefined coarse sea salt
1 quart (or liter) filtered water

In a large, clean crock or a large glass or ceramic bowl, layer the green cabbage, chilis, and garlic until the crock is full or you have used all the ingredients. Using a wooden spoon or your clean fist, push down the cabbage mixture to make it more compact and to release the juices.

In a pitcher or large measuring cup, dissolve the salt in the water, stirring if necessary to encourage the salt to dissolve. Pour the saltwater over the cabbage mixture until the ingredients are submerged, leaving a couple of inches of room at the top for the ingredients to expand.

Place a plate that fits inside the crock or bowl over the cabbage-water mixture, and weigh it down with food-safe weights or a bowl or jar of water, making sure the vegetables remain submerged under the water-salt brine as they ferment. Cover with a lid or cloth, and allow it to ferment for at least two weeks, checking periodically to ensure that the cabbage mixture is still submerged below the water line.

If any mold forms on the surface, simply scoop it out. It will not spoil the sauerkraut unless it gets deeper inside the crock. It may form where the mixture meets the air, but it rarely forms deeper inside the crock.

After two weeks, or longer if you prefer a tangier sauerkraut, dish out the sauerkraut into jars or a bowl, cover, and place in the fridge, where it will usually last for at least a year. Serve topped with slices of the chilis, if desired.

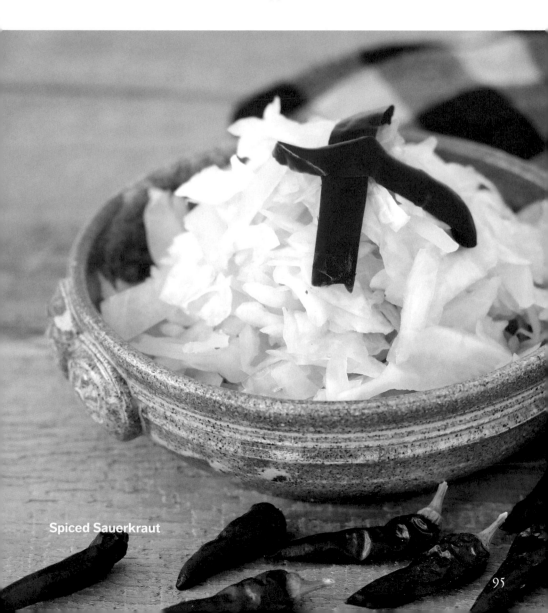

Spiced Sauerkraut

Five-Minute Broccoli Sauerkraut

While it takes at least a week to ferment, I call this "Five-Minute Broccoli Sauerkraut" because it takes only five minutes of preparation time. Even the busiest person can find five minutes to prepare this delicious and healthy sauerkraut. You use a package of broccoli slaw mix found in most grocery stores along with the flavor additions of red pepper and jalapeño. Add a brine, wait a week or two, et voilà! You can eat it over brown rice or noodles, atop salads, on sandwiches or wraps, as a side dish to increase your meals' health factor, or even on its own.

Makes approximately 1 quart

1 (10-ounce or 282-mg) package broccoli coleslaw mix (you don't need the
    packaged dressing if the one you choose contains it)
1 red bell pepper, cored and julienned
1 jalapeño pepper, cored and julienned
3 tablespoons unrefined fine sea salt or 6 tablespoons unrefined coarse sea salt
1 quart (or liter) filtered water

In a large, clean crock or large glass or ceramic bowl, alternate layers of broccoli slaw, bell pepper, and jalapeño pepper inside the crock until the mixture is approximately 1 to 2 inches from the top of the crock or bowl or until you have used all the ingredients. Push the vegetables down with your clean fist or a wooden spoon to release the juices as you go.

In a pitcher or large measuring cup, dissolve the salt in the water, stirring if necessary to encourage the salt to dissolve. Pour the saltwater over the vegetable mixture until the ingredients are submerged, leaving a couple of inches of room at the top for the vegetables to expand.

Place a plate that fits inside the crock or bowl over the vegetable-water mixture, and weigh it down with food-safe weights or a bowl or jar of water, making sure the vegetables remain submerged under the brine as they ferment. (Ideally, choose the biggest plate possible to fit inside the crock and

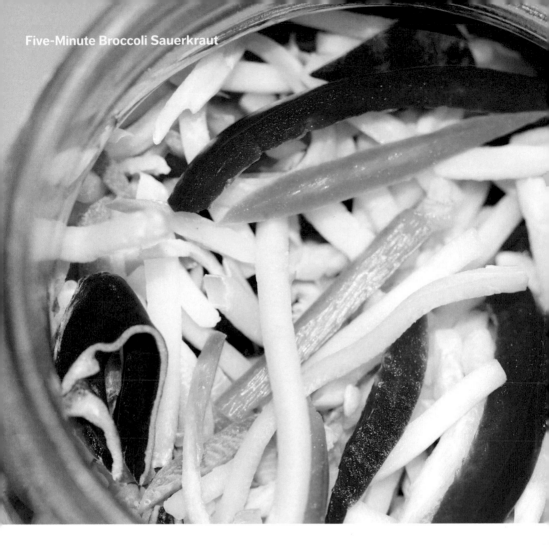

provide the greatest amount of surface coverage to prevent broccoli pieces from floating to the top of the crock.) Cover with a lid or a cloth, and allow it to ferment for at least two weeks, checking periodically to ensure that the cabbage mixture is still submerged below the water line. After two weeks the sauerkraut will still be fairly crunchy; if you like a more traditional sauerkraut, allow it to ferment longer to soften the cabbage further.

If any mold forms on the surface, simply scoop it out. It will not spoil the sauerkraut unless it gets deeper inside the crock. It may form where the mixture meets the air, but it rarely forms deeper inside the crock.

After one week, or longer if you prefer a tarter-tasting sauerkraut, dish out the sauerkraut into jars or a bowl, cover, and place in the fridge, where it will last for at least a few months to a year.

Pineapple Sauerkraut

While this recipe is technically a type of sauerkraut because it is made primarily of shredded cabbage, it has an almost Asian flavor that makes it perfect for serving atop a bowl of brown rice or soba noodles for a quick and healthy rice or noodle bowl meal. Because it contains a whole pineapple, many assume it will be sweet tasting, but depending on the amount of fermentation time, it tends to taste more salty than sweet. It still has a delicious pineapple flavor that works beautifully with the cabbage and carrots. And don't worry if you're not an onion fan: the onion is so mild that even people who don't like onion will probably like this sauerkraut. While I found that I preferred the flavor after two weeks of fermentation time, you can vary it according to your taste, from anywhere between one week and a month. Chop the cabbage as thinly as possible to ensure it ferments sufficiently.

Makes about 3 quarts

1 medium pineapple, top, core, and skin removed (save the scraps if you want to make Pineapple Vinegar, page 138), julienned
1 medium head cabbage, thinly grated
2 medium carrots, grated
¼ small onion, grated
3 tablespoons unrefined fine sea salt or 6 tablespoons unrefined coarse sea salt
2 quarts (or liters) filtered water
Cilantro sprigs for garnish (optional)

In a large, clean 4-quart crock or a large glass or ceramic bowl, alternate layers of pineapple, cabbage, carrots, and onion until the mixture is approximately 1 to 2 inches from the top of the crock or bowl or until you have used all the ingredients. Push down the vegetables with your clean fist or a wooden spoon to release the juices as you go.

In a pitcher or large measuring cup, dissolve the salt in the water, stirring if necessary to encourage the salt to dissolve. Pour the saltwater over the pineapple mixture until the ingredients are submerged, leaving a couple of inches of room at the top for the ingredients to expand.

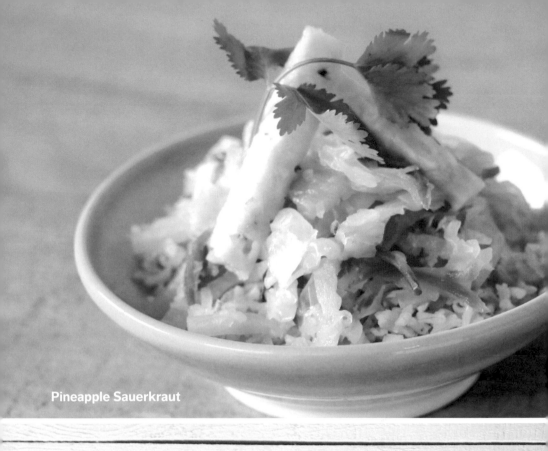

Pineapple Sauerkraut

Place a plate that fits inside the crock or bowl over the pineapple-water mixture, and weigh it down with food-safe weights or a bowl or jar of water, making sure the fruit and vegetables remain submerged under the brine as they ferment. (Ideally, choose the biggest plate possible to fit inside the crock and provide the greatest amount of surface coverage to prevent cabbage pieces from floating to the top of the crock.) Cover with a lid or a cloth, and allow it to ferment for at least two weeks, checking periodically to ensure that the pineapple mixture is still submerged below the water line. After two weeks the sauerkraut will still be fairly crunchy; if you like a more traditional sauerkraut, allow it to ferment longer to soften the cabbage further.

If any mold forms on the surface, simply scoop it out. It will not spoil the sauerkraut unless it gets deeper inside the crock. It may form where the mixture meets the air, but it rarely forms deeper inside the crock.

After two weeks, or longer if you prefer a tangier sauerkraut, dish out the sauerkraut into jars or a bowl, cover, and place in the fridge, where it will last for at least a few months to a year. Serve topped with cilantro sprigs, if desired.

Purple Sauerkraut

This brilliant-colored sauerkraut is as delicious as it is beautiful. It derives its lovely hue from the naturally occurring pigments in purple cabbage, known as proanthocyanidins. During the fermentation process this color transfers from one side of the cabbage to the whole leaf. It's a colorful addition to any meal and is particularly good served on a bed of plain brown rice or noodles.

Makes approximate 2 to 2½ quarts

1 small head green cabbage, shredded
1 small head purple cabbage, shredded
2 apples, thinly sliced
3 tablespoons unrefined fine sea salt or 6 tablespoons unrefined coarse sea salt
1 quart (or liter) filtered water

In a large, clean crock or a large glass or ceramic bowl, layer the green cabbage, purple cabbage, and apples until the mixture is approximately 1 to 2 inches from the top of the crock or bowl or you have used all the ingredients. Push down the cabbage and apple mixture with your clean fist or a wooden spoon to make it more compact and to release the juices as you go.

In a pitcher or large measuring cup, dissolve the salt in the water, stirring if necessary to encourage the salt to dissolve. Pour the saltwater over the cabbage-apple mixture until the ingredients are submerged, leaving a couple of inches of room at the top for the ingredients to expand.

Place a plate that fits inside the crock or bowl over the cabbage-apple-water mixture, and weigh it down with food-safe weights or a bowl or jar of water, making sure the vegetables remain submerged under the brine as they ferment. (Ideally, choose the biggest plate possible to fit inside the crock and provide the greatest amount of surface coverage to prevent cabbage pieces from floating to the top of the crock.) Cover with a lid or a cloth, and allow it to ferment for at least two weeks, checking periodically to ensure that the cabbage-apple mixture is still submerged below the water line. After two weeks the sauerkraut will still be fairly crunchy; if you like a more traditional sauerkraut, allow it to ferment longer to soften the cabbage further.

If any mold forms on the surface, simply scoop it out. It will not spoil the sauerkraut unless it gets deeper inside the crock. It may form where the mixture meets the air, but it rarely forms deeper inside the crock.

After two weeks, or longer if you prefer a tangier sauerkraut, dish out the sauerkraut into jars or a bowl, cover, and place in the fridge, where it will usually last for at least a year.

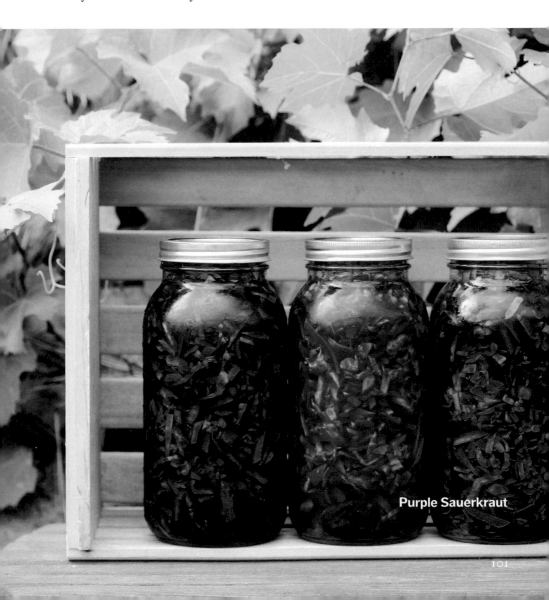

Purple Sauerkraut

Traditionally Fermented Pickles and Vegetable Ferments

Now that you've made your first batch of sauerkraut, you're ready to apply your newfound fermenting skills to make other types of ferments, including traditional pickles. Long before pickles were made by pouring vinegar and spices over vegetables, people used the same brining and submerging processes that brought us sauerkraut. Over the years companies and home cooks opted for using vinegar because the pickles were completed in shorter periods of time; however, the slow food process of making pickles through fermentation is far superior because the flavors develop naturally, resulting in richer-tasting, less acidic pickles than their vinegar-based counterparts. Additionally, vinegar-based pickles offer minimal, if any, nutritional value, while fermented pickles are packed with probiotics.

The process for making pickled vegetables is almost identical to making sauerkraut: simply chop your vegetables and place them in a crock or wide-mouth mason jar, prepare a brine, pour it over the vegetables, place a weight over the vegetables to hold them submerged in the brine, and cover to allow the vegetables to ferment. The only real difference is the type of vegetables used and the shape you chop them. Sauerkrauts are largely shredded cabbage, while pickled vegetables can be any number of vegetables, whether on their own or combined into a mixture. The pickled vegetables can include cabbage, but it's not necessary to use it. You'll also want to add various flavorings to your pickled vegetables, such as herbs and spices, onion and garlic, or chilis to add heat.

You can experiment with a wide variety of vegetable pickles. You'll notice that the cucumbers in my Spicy Dill Fermented Pickles are cut into long slices, while the blend of vegetables in my Taco Pickles are cut into much smaller chunks. Of course, feel free to try whatever suits you best, keeping in mind that you'll need to keep them submerged in the brine, and that may be more difficult with smaller vegetable sizes.

Similar to sauerkraut, you'll need to use sea salt instead of iodized salt, as the iodine prevents the growth of beneficial microorganisms. Let's explore the great world of pickles!

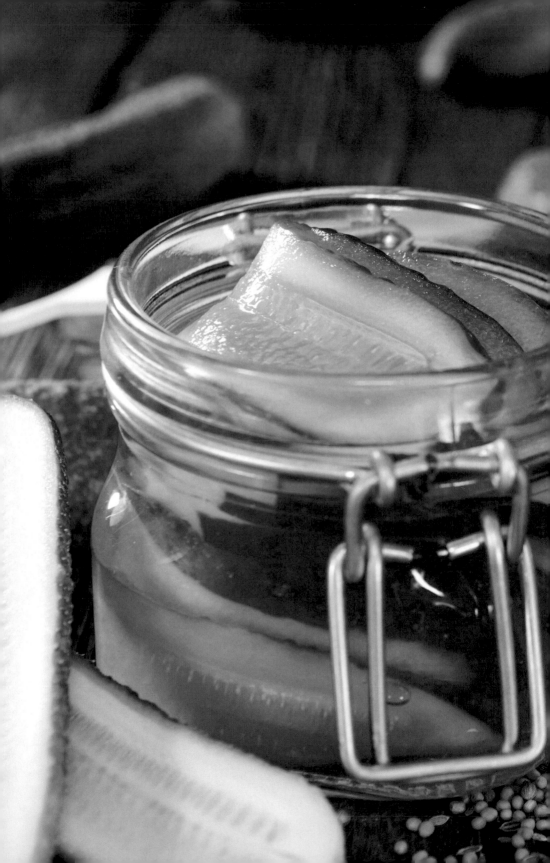

Spicy Dill Fermented Pickles

While most pickles available in grocery stores are made with white vinegar and have few, if any, nutritional benefits, these rely on the traditional method of fermentation to develop the flavors and boost the pickles' probiotic benefits. Once you try these delicious dill pickles and discover how easy they are to make, you'll be happy to leave the store-bought pickles behind.

Makes about 2 quarts

4 large or 6 medium cucumbers or lemon cucumbers, quartered lengthwise
3 dried cayenne chili peppers
2 garlic cloves
4 sprigs fresh dill
3 tablespoons unrefined fine sea salt or 6 tablespoons unrefined coarse sea salt
1½ quarts (or liters) or 6 cups filtered water

In a large, clean crock or a large glass or ceramic bowl, combine the cucumbers, chili peppers, garlic, and dill.

In a pitcher or large measuring cup, dissolve the salt in the water, stirring if necessary to encourage the salt to dissolve. Pour the saltwater over the cucumber mixture until the ingredients are submerged, leaving a couple of inches of room at the top for the ingredients to expand.

Place a plate that fits inside the crock or bowl over the cucumber-water mixture, and weigh it down with food-safe weights or a bowl or jar of water, making sure the vegetables remain submerged under the brine as they ferment. (Ideally, choose the biggest plate possible to fit inside the crock and provide the greatest amount of surface coverage to prevent vegetable pieces from floating to the top of the crock.) Cover with a lid or a cloth, and allow it to ferment for five to seven days, or longer if you prefer a tangier taste; check the mixture periodically to ensure that it is still submerged below the water line.

If any mold forms on the surface, simply scoop it out. It will not spoil the pickles unless it gets deeper inside the crock. It may form where the mixture meets the air, but it rarely forms deeper inside the crock.

After one week, or longer if you prefer a tangier pickle, dish out the pickles into jars or a bowl, cover, and place in the fridge, where they will usually last for up to a year.

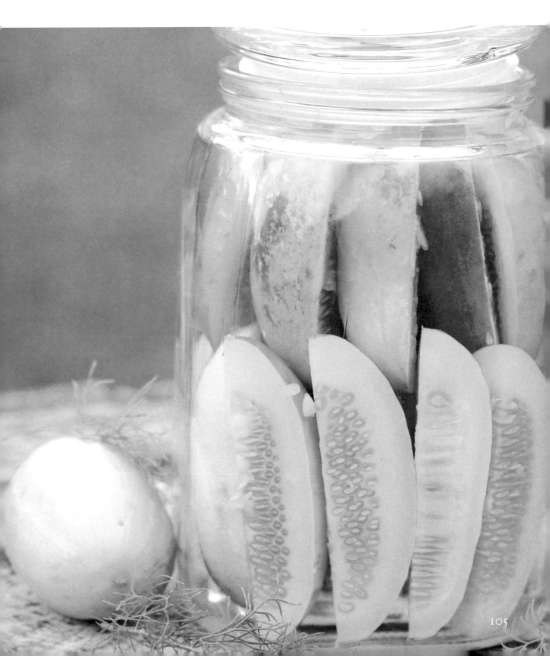

Salvadoran Salsa

This gingery and spicy salsa is one of my favorites. Also known as *curtido*, a traditional Salvadoran fermented salsa-like food, I've given this version a slight twist by adding turmeric and green apple. The result is outstanding. It's great on its own, served as a condiment with chips, on your favorite sausages, or over a salad. You can also mix a couple of heaping spoonfuls with freshly mashed avocado for a new and fermented take on guacamole.

Makes about 1 quart/liter

½ green cabbage
1 to 2 carrots
1 green apple, cored and quartered
One 2-inch piece fresh ginger
½ cayenne chili
½ small purple onion
One 2-inch piece fresh turmeric
3 tablespoons unrefined fine sea salt or 6 tablespoons unrefined coarse sea salt
1 quart (or liter) filtered water

Using a food processor with a coarse grating blade, shred the cabbage, carrots, apple, ginger, chili, onion, and turmeric. (You may wish to use food-safe gloves to avoid touching the chili.) Transfer to a crock or a large glass or ceramic bowl, and mix them together well.

In a pitcher or large measuring cup, dissolve the salt in the water, stirring if necessary to encourage the salt to dissolve. Pour the saltwater over the salsa mixture until the ingredients are submerged, leaving a couple of inches of room at the top for the ingredients to expand.

Place a plate that fits inside the crock or bowl over the salsa-water mixture, and weigh it down with food-safe weights or a bowl or jar of water, making sure the vegetables remain submerged under the brine as they ferment. (Ideally, choose the biggest plate possible to fit inside the crock and

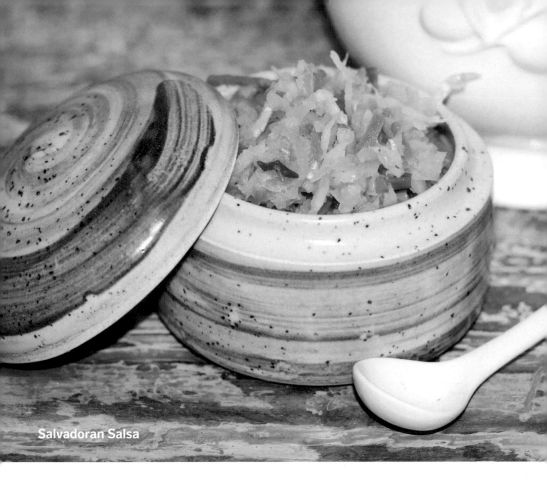

Salvadoran Salsa

provide the greatest amount of surface coverage to prevent vegetable pieces from floating to the top of the crock.) Cover with a lid or a cloth, and allow it to ferment for five to seven days, checking periodically to ensure that the salsa mixture is still submerged below the water line.

If any mold forms on the surface, simply scoop it out. It will not spoil the salsa unless it gets deeper inside the crock. It may form where the mixture meets the air, but it rarely forms deeper inside the crock.

After one week, dish out the salsa into jars or a bowl, cover, and place in the fridge, where it will usually last up to one year.

Star Anise Carrots

I love the licorice-type flavor of star anise combined with carrots. During fermentation the carrots pick up the delicate flavor along with a slight sour note from the culturing process. These pickles are delicious on their own, alongside your meal to add an extra vegetable, or inside wraps.

Makes about 1 quart/liter

1½ pounds carrots, grated
3 whole star anise pods
3 tablespoons unrefined fine sea salt or 6 tablespoons unrefined coarse sea salt
1 quart (or liter) filtered water

In a medium, clean crock or a medium glass or ceramic bowl, combine the carrots and star anise.

In a pitcher or large measuring cup, dissolve the salt in the water, stirring if necessary to encourage the salt to dissolve. Pour the saltwater over the carrot mixture until the ingredients are submerged, leaving a couple of inches of room at the top for the ingredients to expand.

Place a plate that fits inside the crock or bowl over the carrot-water mixture, and weigh it down with food-safe weights or a bowl or jar of water, making sure the carrots remain submerged under the brine as they ferment. (Ideally, choose the biggest plate possible to fit inside the crock and provide the greatest amount of surface coverage to prevent carrot pieces from floating to the top of the crock.) Cover with a lid or a cloth, and allow it to ferment for seven days, checking periodically to ensure that the carrot mixture is still submerged below the water line.

If any mold forms on the surface, simply scoop it out. It will not spoil the carrots unless it gets deeper inside the crock. It may form where the mixture meets the air, but it rarely forms deeper inside the crock.

After one week, dish out the carrots into jars or a bowl, cover, and place in the fridge, where it will usually last up to one year.

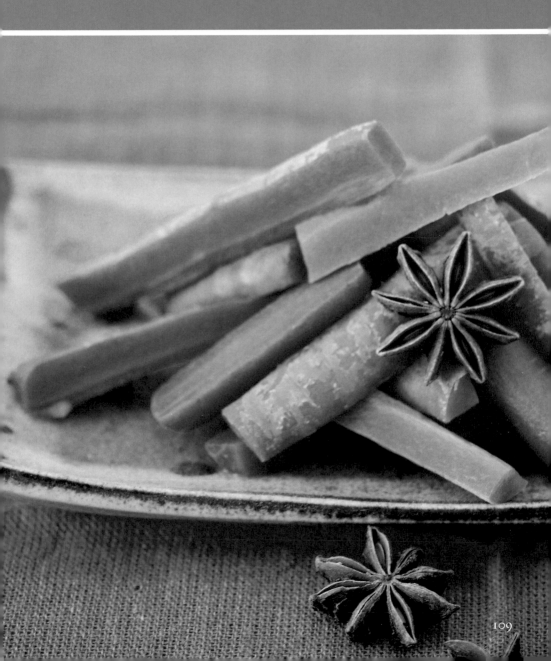

Cultured Onions

I know cultured onions may not make your top-ten list of recipes you wish to make, but I encourage you to make them anyway. The culturing process mellows the onions' flavor, making them a versatile and delicious addition to wraps, sandwiches, or salads. I'm not a big fan of raw onions, but I love cultured onions, particularly on Greek or Middle Eastern–inspired wrap sandwiches. Plus, they're practical to keep on hand when you want to add a slight onion flavor to a dish but don't feel like chopping a whole onion.

Makes about 2 cups

2 small onions or 1 large onion, chopped into thin slices
1 tablespoon plus 1 teaspoon unrefined fine sea salt
1 cup filtered water

Place the onions in a small sealable jar. In a measuring cup, dissolve the salt in the water, stirring if necessary to encourage the salt to dissolve. Pour the saltwater over the onions in the jar until the ingredients are submerged, leaving some room at the top for the onions to expand.

Weigh down with a small ramekin, food-safe weight, or fermentation weights. Cover with a lid or a cloth, and allow it to ferment for two to seven days. Shorter fermentation times result in stronger onions, and longer fermentation times mellow out the oniony taste and increase the probiotic content. After your desired fermentation time, remove the weights, seal, and store in the refrigerator, where the onions will usually last up to a year.

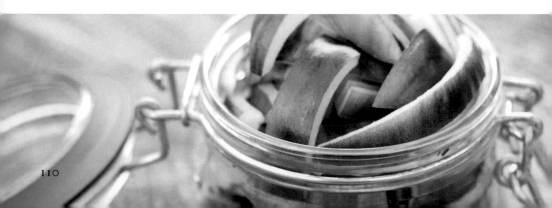

Red-Hot Hot Sauce

I love adding a splash of heat to almost everything I eat. It's not uncommon to see my eyes well up with tears while eating, and although occasionally this may be due to the overwhelmingly delicious taste, more often it is because I've turned up the heat on my meals with a splash of red-hot hot sauce.

Makes about 2 to 3 cups

1 pound red chilis (use whatever type you'd like: Thai, habaneros, cayenne, etc., keeping in mind that the type of chilis used will determine the heat level of the final sauce)
4 tablespoons unrefined fine sea salt or 8 tablespoons unrefined coarse sea salt
5 cups filtered water

Wash the chilis and place them in a glass or ceramic jar with a wide opening or in a bowl.

In a pitcher or large measuring cup, dissolve the salt in the water, stirring if necessary to encourage the salt to dissolve. Pour the saltwater over the chilis until they are submerged, leaving a couple of inches of room at the top for the ingredients to expand.

Place a plate that fits inside the jar or bowl over the chili-water mixture, and weigh it down with food-safe weights or a small bowl or jar of water, making sure the chilis remain submerged under the brine as they ferment.

Cover with a lid or a cloth, and allow it to ferment for seven days, checking periodically to ensure that the chilis are still submerged below the water line. Strain off the brine, reserving it to add, as needed, to the chilis to obtain your desired hot-sauce consistency.

Place the chilis in a blender, and blend with enough brine to get a slightly thinner hot sauce than you would like; it will thicken as it sits. Pour into a jar or bowl, cover, and refrigerate, where it should last about one month.

See photo on page 82.

Fermented Chopped Salad

We all know we should eat more salads, but let's face it: sometimes it feels like too much work to chop all those vegetables. I created the fermented chopped salad so you only need to chop once and can eat many times. Because it stores for many months in the fridge, I can have an easy salad on those lazy, hazy days when I need more vegetables but don't want to do the work. It is great on its own but can also be tossed in a vinaigrette or served over a bowl of brown rice for a quick and easy, delicious and nutritious rice bowl dinner.

Makes about 6 cups

1 radish, finely chopped
½ small onion, finely chopped
1 turnip, chopped in ½-inch chunks
1 carrot, chopped in ½-inch chunks
3 small apples, chopped in ½-inch chunks
Handful of green beans, chopped in 1-inch lengths
1 rutabaga, chopped in ½-inch chunks
1 to 2 grape leaves, kale leaves, or other large leafy greens (optional)
3 tablespoons unrefined fine sea salt or 6 tablespoons unrefined coarse sea salt
1 quart (or liter) filtered water

In a medium bowl, toss together the radish, onion, turnip, carrot, apples, green beans, and rutabaga; transfer to a small crock. Place the grape leaves or other leafy greens over the top of the chopped salad ingredients to help hold them under the brine, and weigh down with food-safe weights or a jar or bowl of water.

In a pitcher or large measuring cup, dissolve the salt in the water, stirring if necessary to encourage the salt to dissolve. Pour the brine over the salad, cover with a lid or cloth, and allow it to ferment for one week. Remove the weights, and remove and discard the grape leaves or other leafy greens. Dish out to jars or a bowl, cover, and refrigerate, where the salad should last six months to one year.

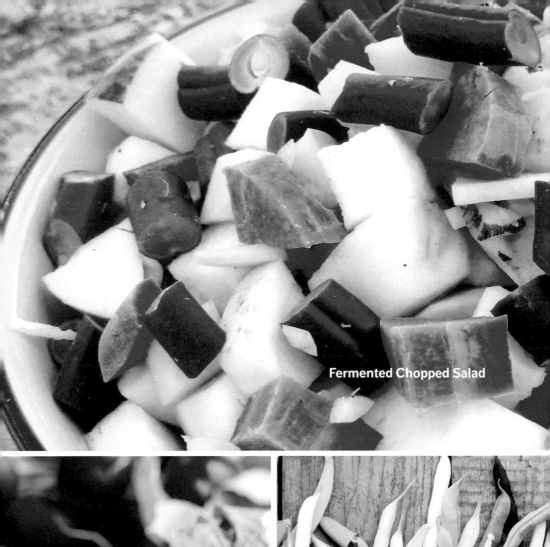
Fermented Chopped Salad

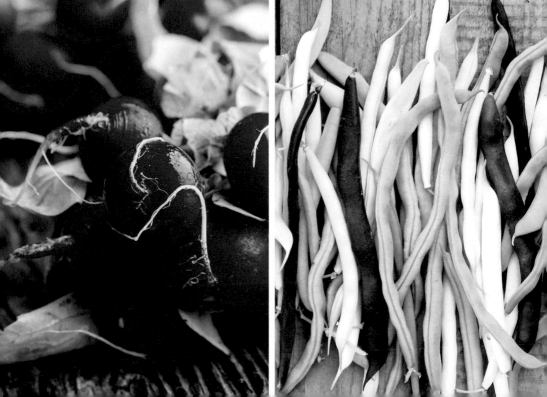

Dill Cucumber Pickle Bites

We live on a mountainside, so we have terraced gardens. I decided last year to turn one of the stone walls into a squash and cucumber wall by planting the vegetable seeds in the garden bed above and letting the plants trail down the wall. The idea was a huge success. Before I knew it we had over twenty feet of squashes and cucumbers growing down the six- to seven-foot wall — and, as you can imagine, more cucumbers than we knew what to do with. After juicing them as well as eating plentiful amounts of Greek salad and Tzatziki (see recipe on page 160), I turned my attention to pickling them. I thought it would be great to have smaller-sized pickles as a side dish to many summer meals or autumn and winter soups and sandwiches, so I made these pickle bites. They're simple to make, and once you've tried them, you'll want to make them a regular part of your fermentation regime.

Makes about 4 cups

1 large cucumber, or 2–3 lemon cucumbers, chopped into 1-inch to 2-inch chunks
2 to 3 medium sprigs fresh dill
3 tablespoons unrefined fine sea salt or 6 tablespoons unrefined coarse sea salt
1 quart (or liter) filtered water

Place the cucumbers in a large mason jar, interspersing dill sprigs throughout as you go. Weigh down the cucumbers with a food-safe clean weight inside the mason jar.

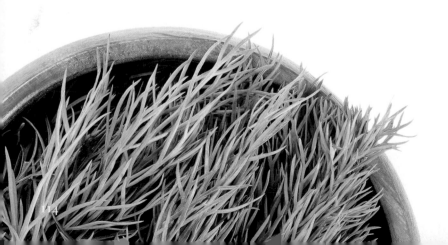

In a pitcher or large measuring cup, dissolve the salt in the water, stirring if necessary to encourage the salt to dissolve. Pour the saltwater over the cucumbers until they are submerged, leaving some room at the top for the ingredients to expand. Cover with a lid, and allow it to ferment for five to seven days, or until the cucumbers have reached your desired tanginess.

Remove the weights, replace the cover, and refrigerate, where the pickles will last for six months to one year.

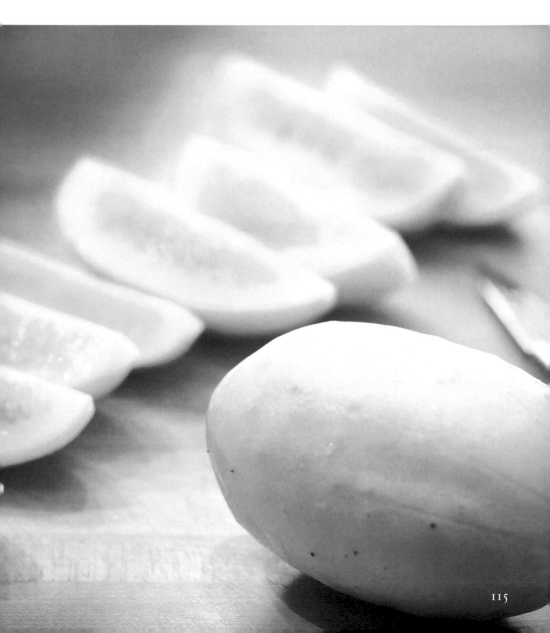

Zucchini Pickles

Like their cucumber counterparts, zucchini pickles are easy to make and even easier to eat. Curtis and I grew zucchini from seed last year. At first it looked like only one seed grew into a plant, but then another couple of plants unexpectedly reared their heads. By the end of summer I could no longer keep up with the dozens of zucchini coming up in the garden, so I decided to try making zucchini pickles. I even made them with a couple of oversized zucchinis that had fairly tough skins and were considered largely inedible. To my surprise, the fermentation processes softened the skins, and the resulting pickles were delicious. Of course, if you're trying this recipe with marrow zucchini with seriously thick and hard skins, it may not work, so do so at your own risk. But this recipe works very well with softer-skinned zucchinis and is a great way to use up any summer stash you might have.

Makes about 8 cups

½ teaspoon whole coriander seeds
½ dried cayenne chili, crushed
2 whole cloves
½ teaspoon anise seeds
½ teaspoon mustard seeds
½ teaspoon ground turmeric
¼ teaspoon ground pepper
2 large or 4 small zucchinis, cut into 1-inch chunks or long, thin spears, approximately
   3 inches long, ½ inch across
3 tablespoons unrefined fine sea salt or 6 tablespoons unrefined coarse sea salt
2 quarts (or liters) filtered water

Combine the coriander, chili, cloves, anise, mustard, turmeric, and pepper in a small to medium crock. Add the zucchini and stir to combine. Weigh down the zucchini with clean, food-safe weights or a jar or bowl of water.

In a pitcher or large measuring cup, dissolve the salt in the water, stirring if necessary to encourage the salt to dissolve. Pour the saltwater into

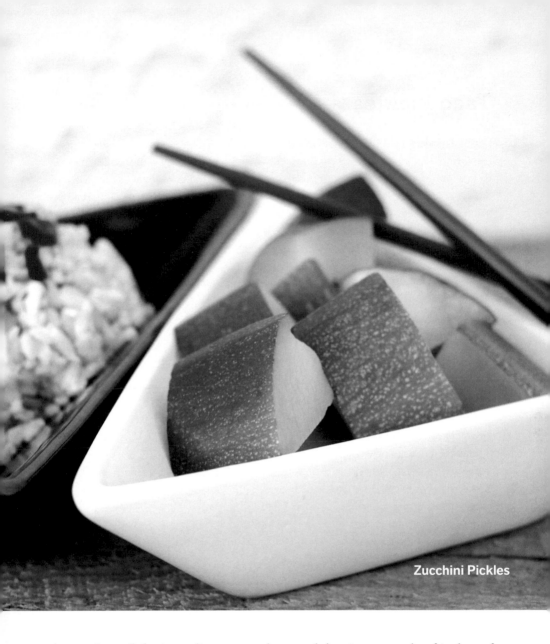

Zucchini Pickles

the crock until the ingredients are submerged, leaving a couple of inches of room at the top for the ingredients to expand.

Cover with a lid or a cloth, and allow it to ferment for five to seven days, or until it has reached your desired tanginess. Remove the weights, dish out into jars or a bowl, cover, and refrigerate, where the pickles should last for six months to one year.

Taco Pickles

I call this recipe *Taco Pickles* because the vegetables are chopped finely enough to fit comfortably within a hard taco shell, and the flavors pair perfectly with taco filling ingredients. But to be honest, I eat these more on their own than I do with tacos because they are just so delicious. No matter how big of a batch I make, I always run out before I can get another one made. They are delicious served with all types of Mexican or Tex-Mex foods, like burritos, enchiladas, tacos, and more. They are also good served over brown rice, quinoa, or noodles for a quick rice or noodle bowl meal. The first time I created these pickles I was instantly addicted, and now they are one of my favorite fermented foods. Curtis even wondered aloud, "How can raw cauliflower taste this good?" when he eats my taco pickles.

Makes about 1 quart/liter

½ medium cauliflower, coarsely chopped into about nickel-size pieces
¼ cabbage, coarsely chopped
1 medium carrot, coarsely chopped
½ jalapeño pepper, finely chopped
¼ red bell pepper, coarsely chopped
½ stalk celery, coarsely chopped
1 tablespoon turmeric powder
1 quart (or liter) filtered water
3 tablespoons unrefined fine sea salt or 6 tablespoons unrefined coarse sea salt

In a small to medium crock, combine the cauliflower, cabbage, carrot, jalapeño, bell pepper, and celery, and toss until they are well mixed.

In a small bowl or pitcher, mix together the turmeric powder, water, and salt until the sea salt has dissolved. Pour the saltwater mixture over the chopped vegetables until the ingredients are submerged, leaving a couple of inches of room at the top for the ingredients to expand. Weight the vegetables with clean, food-safe weights or a jar or bowl of water to keep the vegetables submerged. Cover with a lid or a cloth, and allow it to ferment for five days.

Remove the weights, transfer the vegetables and some brine to jars or a bowl, cover, and refrigerate, where it should last for up to a year.

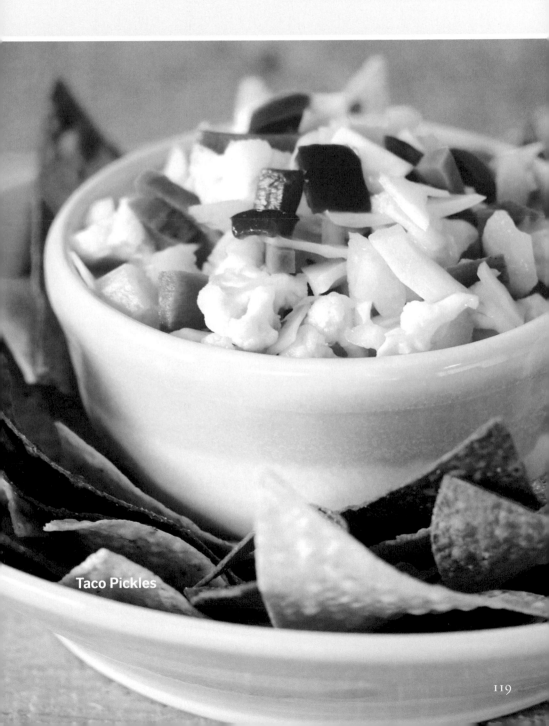

Taco Pickles

Kimchi: The Fermented Food That Helps Protect against Dementia

When we think of dementia — or the loss of memory typically associated with aging — most of us don't think of fermented foods. But probiotic-rich foods may play an important role in preventing and even treating this degenerative brain disease.

For many years science led us to believe that we had little control over our brain health and its functioning. Dementia was thought to be the inevitable result of aging. But there is a growing body of research linking what we eat, how we live, how stressed we are, and how much we challenge ourselves intellectually to our overall brain health.

While many people may be aware that purple grapes, blueberries, walnuts, or flax seeds are brain-boosting foods, few know that one particular fermented food stands out as a brain health superfood. No, it's not yogurt — although yogurt with live probiotic cultures may be beneficial to the brain as well. The brain-booster extraordinaire may come as a surprise: kimchi. Kimchi is a fermented blend of cabbage, garlic, onions or scallions, ginger, red pepper or chili peppers, and sometimes other flavor additions that is eaten as an appetizer or condiment.

Scientists have identified a whopping 970 different bacterial strains in kimchi.[5] Compare that to the one, two, or occasionally three strains of probiotics found in most brands of yogurt. Of course, not all kimchis have that many different strains. One strain in particular commonly found in kimchi, *Lactobacillus plantarum*, is a research-proven antioxidant. The brain is quite vulnerable to free radical damage that occurs as we age, eat harmful foods or beverages, and are exposed to harmful substances in the air we breathe or if we experience traumatic brain injuries. Free radicals are unstable molecules that can damage healthy cells and tissues, but antioxidants neutralize free radicals, preventing them from damaging healthy cells in the brain. In a study published in the online medical journal *PLoS One*, *Lactobacillus plantarum* demonstrated antioxidant activity stronger than other probiotics.[6]

In a study published in the *Journal of Applied Microbiology*, researchers tested probiotics extracted from kimchi. One of the probiotics, *Lactobacillus pentosus var. plantarum C29*, showed a potent ability to protect the brain against memory loss. And you don't have to remember its name to benefit from its memory-protective effects: kimchi is the only source of this particular probiotic strain (that I am aware of). The scientists concluded that kimchi and this probiotic "may be beneficial for dementia."[7]

Obviously, more research needs to be conducted, but considering that there are no known side effects other than additional health benefits of eating it, I consider kimchi a great dietary addition, especially if you are experiencing memory issues or are trying to prevent them. In a study published in the *Journal of Medicinal Food*, kimchi was also shown to reduce cholesterol levels and obesity and have anticancer effects, among other benefits.[8]

Not all kimchi is created equally, however. If you are buying your kimchi at a store, be sure to choose one that contains live cultures and has not been pasteurized. You should find it in the refrigerator section of your health food or grocery store. Organic options are best, as pesticides used on crops significantly reduce the beneficial bacterial counts in fermented foods. Better yet, make your own delicious, probiotic-rich kimchi at home. Following is my recipe for White Kimchi — one of my favorite types.

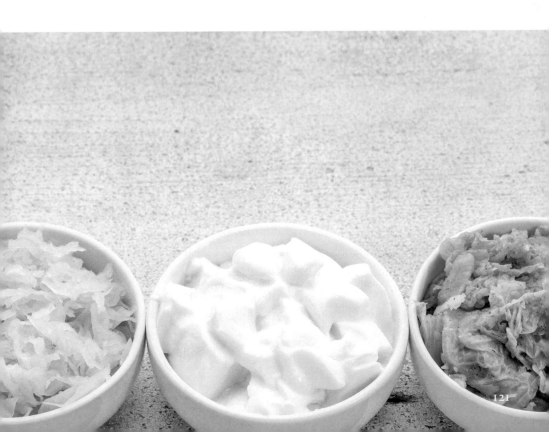

White Kimchi

According to my Korean Canadian friend and avid kimchi maker Bonah, there are over two hundred varieties of kimchi. Because she regularly shares her wonderful kimchi creations with me, I quickly learned about the diverse flavors and kinds of kimchi. One of the first types of kimchi she shared with me lacked the signature reddish color I was accustomed to but had all the great flavor of kimchi that I love. She told me it was a type of kimchi known as *white kimchi*. I've created here a simplified version that has lots of flavor without the heat often associated with kimchi, for those who can't eat spicy foods or anyone looking to try a diverse range of kimchis. Instead of the traditional Korean ingredients, which can be difficult to find in the small town in which I live (and perhaps where you live too), I substituted vegetables that are more readily available.

Makes about 4 quarts

1 large Napa cabbage (about 2½ pounds), quartered, with the stalk removed, and cut into 1-inch chunks
1 large carrot, julienned into 2-inch-long strips
1 large black Spanish radish or 3 red radishes, julienned
1 red bell pepper, seeded, cored, and julienned
3 sprigs green onion or chives, chopped into 1-inch pieces
2 pears (I use red pears, but you can use whatever type is available), stemmed, seeded, and quartered
3 garlic cloves, peeled
½ small onion, quartered
1-inch piece fresh ginger
3 tablespoons unrefined fine sea salt or 6 tablespoons unrefined coarse sea salt
6 cups filtered water

In a large bowl, combine the cabbage, carrot, radish, bell pepper, and green onions.

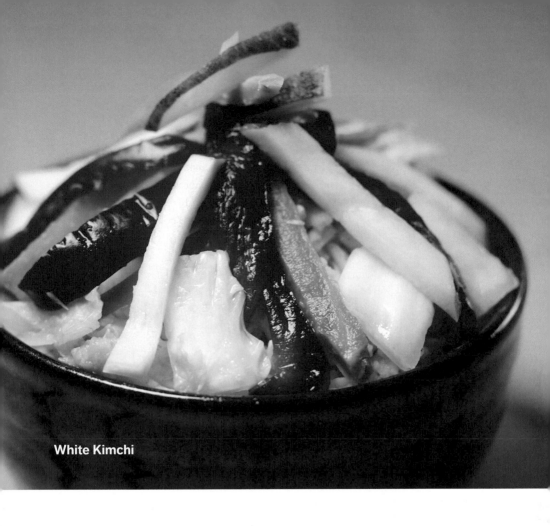

White Kimchi

Combine the pears, garlic, onion, and ginger in a food processor, and blend into a puree. Pour the pear mixture over the chopped vegetables. Add the salt, and toss all the vegetables together until they are evenly coated in the pear puree and salt.

Place the vegetable mixture in a large crock, and pour the water over it. Place a plate that fits inside the crock to cover the vegetables and hold them submerged. Place food-safe weights or a glass bowl or jar filled with water on top of the plate to keep the vegetables submerged. Cover with a lid and store in a cool, undisturbed place for approximately one week or until it has reached your desired level of tanginess.

Transfer to jars or a bowl, cover, and refrigerate, where the kimchi should last for up to a year.

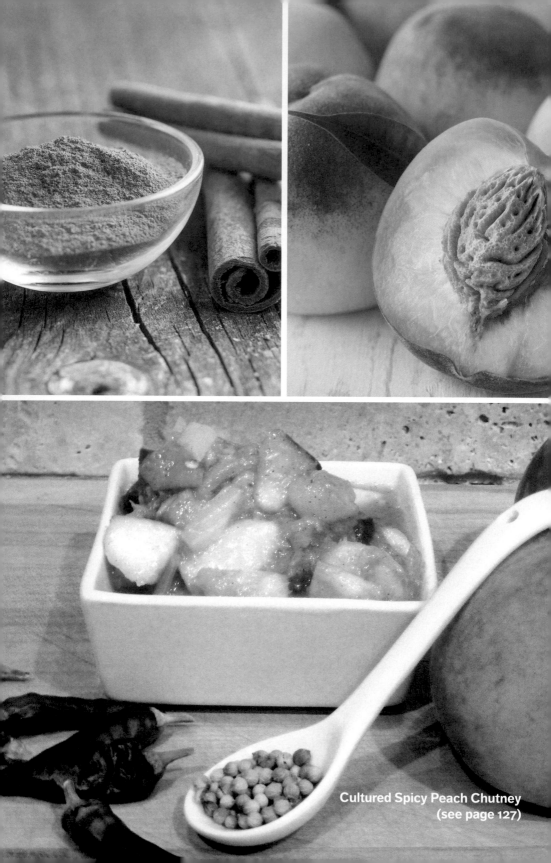

Cultured Spicy Peach Chutney
(see page 127)

CHAPTER FIVE

FRUIT CULTURES AND HOMEMADE VINEGARS

When I first started fermenting foods I didn't give the idea of fermenting fruit much thought. At that time most of the fermented foods I knew about or had eaten were made with vegetables, like sauerkraut and pickles. But as I learned more and my experimentation grew, so did my use of fruit in my ferments. I have since developed many delightful fruit ferments, some of which are among my all-time favorite fermented foods.

While many of the fermentation processes for fruits are similar to those used for vegetables, there are some variations. For example, using a saltwater solution — a brine — is not as common with fruit as it is with vegetables. It's not that you can't brine fruit, but doing so will cause it to lose a significant amount of its natural sweetness. And fruit can be added to many vegetable ferments (you'll notice numerous recipes that use both fruit and vegetables in chapter 4). I encourage you to try fermenting a wide range of fruits and vegetables or combinations. But I also urge you to try many of the lightly fermented foods I include in this chapter. By *lightly fermented* I mean shortened fermentation times — sometimes overnight or for a single day. Of course, when it comes to making vinegar out of fruit, the fermentation time takes a little longer. Regardless of whether your fermentation is short or long, fermenting still adds probiotics and nutritional value to your final food products.

Many fruits are fermented in a sugar-water solution instead of a brine. Much of the sugar becomes food (prebiotics) for the naturally occurring microbes, and this promotes the fermentation.

Leftover whey from making yogurt, using the traditional method of separating curds and whey, can also be used to ferment fruit. Simply add two or three tablespoons to the fruit of your choice, cover, and allow it to sit for about twelve hours. Then refrigerate your fruit ferment, and use within four days. These types of ferments don't tend to last as long as those made in a brine or sugar-water solution, but they are quick to make and a delicious way to glean the health benefits of probiotics.

The contents of probiotic capsules, or probiotic powder, can also be used to ferment fruit. Simply empty the contents of one or two capsules or add a half-teaspoon or teaspoon of your favorite probiotic powder to your favorite fruit or fruit combination. Cover and let sit for about twelve hours. Refrigerate and use within four days. I suggest using a probiotic powder that doesn't contain beneficial yeasts (usually they start with *Saccharomyces* on the ingredient list, or sometimes it is shortened to *S.*) because the yeasts can give your ferment a less-than-desirable taste.

There are advantages to fermenting fruit. For example, many fruits like grapes, apples, or blueberries, among others, have a whitish substance coating them. That is a built-in probiotic starter culture known as a *bloom*. Like me, you probably washed or wiped it off your fruit. Although I still encourage you to wash the fruit you use, try to maintain the inherent bloom on these foods, as it makes them perfect for culturing.

In this chapter you'll learn some of the basic fruit fermentation processes and discover my favorite fermented fruit recipes:

- Cultured Spicy Peach Chutney
- Sweet Vanilla Peaches
- Crabapple Vinegar
- Apple Vinegar
- Apple Cider Vinegar
- Pineapple Vinegar

Cultured Spicy Peach Chutney

Curtis and I have three mature peach trees in our yard. At the end of June or early July these trees begin to burst forth their bounty in sweet, juicy peaches. For about a month we enjoy peaches fresh from the tree, and we add them to curries, salads, and ice tea. But inevitably we always end up with more peaches than we know what to do with, so I began fermenting them. I came up with this deliciously sweet and spicy peach chutney, which we polished off in a day. So I tripled the recipe to make enough for the week. It is delicious on yogurt, on your favorite hot dogs or sausage (including vegan options), or served with roasted vegetables or along with your favorite curry dish. I particularly love it with chickpea curries. If you prefer a less spicy chutney, just omit or reduce the amount of the cayenne chili.

Makes approximately 2 to 3 cups

½ small onion, chopped (about ⅓ cup chopped) and sautéed
2 medium peaches, pitted and coarsely chopped
½ teaspoon unrefined sea salt
Pinch black pepper
⅛ teaspoon cloves
¼ teaspoon turmeric powder
½ teaspoon ground coriander
½ teaspoon cinnamon
1 cayenne pepper, dried and crushed
3 tablespoons whey, 2 probiotic capsules, or ½ teaspoon probiotic powder

Combine all the ingredients in a bowl; if you're using probiotic capsules, empty the contents into the fruit mixture, and discard the empty capsule shells. Toss until it is mixed well. Pour the mixture into a half-quart (500 mL) mason jar with a lid, cover, and leave at room temperature for approximately twelve hours. Refrigerate, where it should keep for about four days.

See photo on page 124.

Sweet Vanilla Peaches

This recipe, which is my favorite ice cream topper, evolved from our abundant peach supply one summer. Because we have so many of these delicious fruits, I was searching for new ways to incorporate them into our diet. And so the idea of fermented sweet vanilla peaches sprung forth. They are superb on their own or make a delicious topping for ice cream, pudding, toast, oatmeal, or brown rice cereal.

Makes about 5 cups

5 medium peaches, pitted and coarsely chopped (about 5 cups chopped)
½ teaspoon vanilla powder
½ teaspoon cardamom powder (optional)
1 tablespoon pure maple syrup
2 tablespoons whey

In a large bowl, combine all the ingredients and mix well. Scoop the mixture into a 1-quart mason jar, cover, and let sit for twelve hours. Refrigerate, where it should keep for four days.

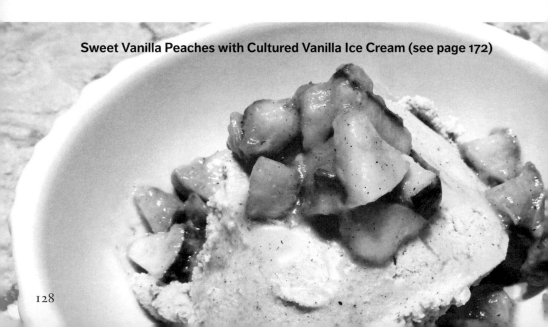

Sweet Vanilla Peaches with Cultured Vanilla Ice Cream (see page 172)

Crabapple Vinegar

Curtis and I have this beautiful crabapple tree in our front yard. Every spring it bursts with stunning pink flowers so thick that the tree looks like one giant pink ball of flowers on a tree trunk. I can't help but smile every time I pass by. By summer it is bursting with thousands of scarlet red crabapples. Instead of letting them find their way onto the lawn and then getting shoveled into the compost, I decided that this year I was going to find a practical use, outside of soil enhancement alone, for these tart fruits.

This was the first time I made vinegar from scratch. I've made infused vinegars before — you know the kind: you pour vinegar over fruit or herbs and strain it in a week or two. But making vinegar from scratch seemed a much more daunting task. What a pleasant surprise to learn that it was so simple. I encourage you to make your own vinegar. When you make it yourself, it's not the lifeless stuff that most store-bought vinegar is: homemade vinegar is packed with beneficial probiotics that boost digestion and add a wonderful flavor to the food you make with it.

The process may seem a bit daunting…particularly when it starts to give off a funky odor partway through the fermentation process. It may be tempting to throw the whole thing out, but if you stick with it, you'll end up with a sweet-tart vinegar that has wonderful flavor nuances and makes a great addition to salads, marinades, and soups.

I made this vinegar with crabapples mostly because I couldn't bear the thought of these lovely little fruits going to waste, but you can use whatever type of fruit you want. The opportunities are really endless here — apple, pineapple, grape, cherry, or whatever type you prefer. While I haven't tried citrus fruits like oranges, kumquats, or grapefruit, I know their peels contain potent antibacterial compounds, so if you want to give them a go, you'll need to peel them first. If you're making vinegar from fruit larger than crabapples, you'll need to cut it into smaller pieces first (about one-inch cubes work well). For crabapples it is as easy as washing and using the fruit whole.

I call for coconut sugar in this recipe, but any type of unrefined sweetener will do — Sucanat, unrefined cane sugar, maple syrup, or honey. Do not use Splenda, NutraSweet, Aminosweet, or other type of artificial sweetener. And although stevia is a natural sweetener, it won't work for making vinegar because it doesn't contain any sugar; it just naturally tastes sweet. You need the sugar to feed the probiotic cultures captured from the fruit and air, and as a natural preservative, preventing mold growth on the fruit as it ferments.

In my directions I've indicated that you need to stir your apple-sugar-water solution every day. This is imperative to ensure that your fruit ferments don't go moldy. I find it best to mark the start and end dates on a calendar so I don't lose track, particularly when I'm making a lot of different cultured foods simultaneously.

Makes about 1 quart/liter

½ cup coconut sugar
1 quart (or liter) filtered water
About 2 pounds crabapples (or enough to fill a 1-quart jar with about 1 inch of space
  remaining), well cleaned

In a pitcher or large measuring cup, mix together the sugar and water, stirring if necessary to encourage the sugar to dissolve.

Place the crabapples in a thoroughly cleaned 1-quart jar with a wide mouth, leaving about 1 inch at the top of the jar. Pour the sugar-water solution over the crabapples, leaving about ¾ inch at the top of the jar. The crabapples will float to the top, and some won't be submerged, but that's okay. Cover the opening with a few layers of clean cheesecloth, and attach an elastic band around the mouth of the jar or crock to hold the cheesecloth in place.

Every day, remove the cheesecloth and stir to cover the crabapples with the sugar-water solution, re-covering with the cheesecloth when you're done. This *must* be done every day to ensure that the apples don't go moldy during the fermentation process.

After two weeks, strain off the crabapples, reserving the liquid; you can add the crabapples to your compost. Pour the liquid into a bottle, and seal with a tight-fitting lid or cork. The vinegar keeps for approximately one year.

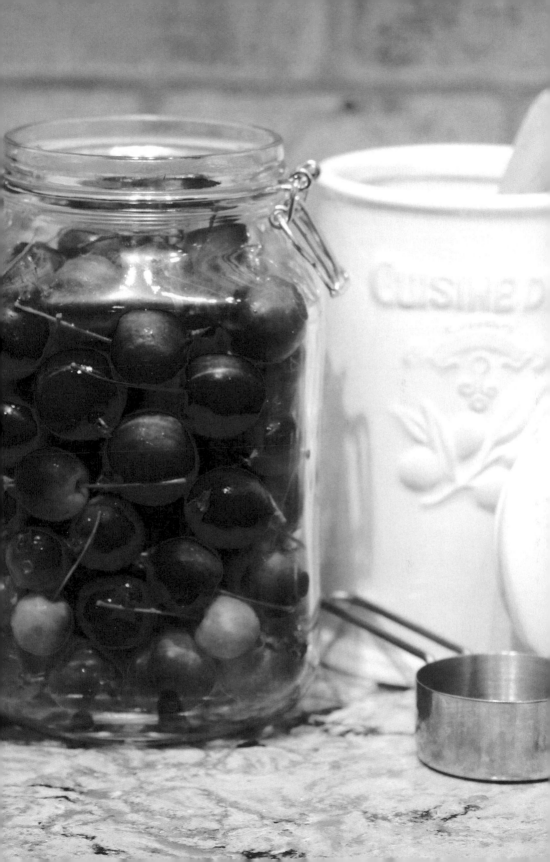

Apple Vinegar

Don't throw away those apples that are spongy and past their prime or the peels and cores from making your favorite apple dishes! You can quickly give these castoffs new life as delicious and nutritious apple vinegar. After I made a successful batch of it, I was hooked. How could it be so simple to turn less-than-desirable fruit and fruit scraps into vinegar? With minimal effort and a minor time and cost investment, the simple process provides delicious, health-building vinegar in a couple of weeks. You'll notice there is sugar in this recipe. It acts as a natural preservative so the apples don't just rot, and it provides food to encourage the growth of probiotic cultures. Apples aren't high in natural sugars, so without the added sugar, they would just grow mold and other unwanted microbes. But don't worry: the beneficial bacteria eat most of the sugar, causing them to multiply as they go. The result: high quantities of beneficial, health-building bacteria.

Makes about ½ to 1 quart/liter

½ cup coconut sugar
1 quart filtered water
4 apples, cores and skins included

In a pitcher or large measuring cup, mix together the sugar and water, stirring if necessary to encourage the sugar to dissolve.

Chop the apples into quarters, and then chop each piece in half. Place the apple pieces, cores and skins included, in a 1- to 2-quart jar or crock, leaving about 1 to 2 inches at the top of the jar.

Pour the sugar-water solution over the apples, leaving about ¾ inch at the top of the jar. The apples will float to the top, and some won't be submerged, but that's okay.

Cover the opening with a few layers of clean cheesecloth, and attach an elastic band around the mouth of the jar or crock to hold the cheesecloth in place.

Every day, remove the cheesecloth, and stir to cover the apples with the sugar-water solution, re-covering with the cheesecloth when you're done. You *must* do this every day to ensure that the apples don't go moldy during the fermentation process.

After two weeks, strain off the apples, reserving the liquid; you can add the apples to your compost. Pour the liquid into a bottle, and seal with a tight-fitting lid or cork. The vinegar keeps for approximately one year.

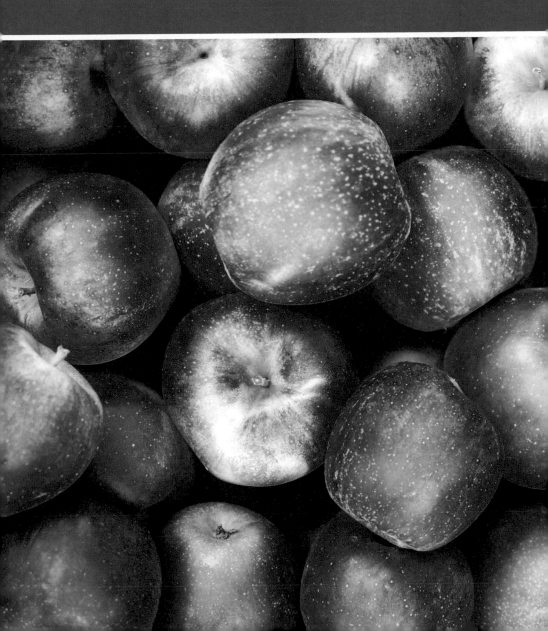

Apple Cider Vinegar

Apple cider vinegar is one of the staples in my home. I use it to preserve freshly harvested herbs and to add flavor to soups, stews, tofu (organic, of course!), and salad dressings. With some olive oil and a teaspoon of crushed chili and basil, I have an absolutely delicious instant bread dip.

While it is possible to buy apple cider vinegar from the local health food or grocery store, it is so simple to make your own, and there is no comparison when it comes to the taste of freshly made apple cider vinegar. Making your own also allows you to control the balance of acidity to sweetness, which you simply cannot do with the store-bought varieties. Once you've made your first apple cider vinegar, you'll probably understand why I insist on making my own.

Making any type of homemade fruit vinegar is as simple as mashing up fruit, removing the pulp, bottling, and leaving it to sit until bacteria known as *Acetobacter* convert the juice into vinegar.

You can also purchase apple cider or apple juice, if you prefer; if you do so, simply skip the juicing step. Here's how to get started making your own apple cider vinegar.

Save up any apples that are beyond their prime. Not rotten ones, of course, but pulpy or spongy apples that are no longer suitable for eating are great for making vinegar. Of course, you can use fresh apples that are absolutely perfect too, but I find that making apple cider vinegar from older apples is the perfect way to use up older ones without sending them to the compost bin. Push them through an electric juicer to make apple juice. If you don't have a juicer, just cut the apples into quarters and puree them in a food processor (you can leave the cores and skins on). Then push the apple pulp through a muslin-lined sieve or muslin bag to remove the fiber from the juice.

Pour the juice into clean, dark, glass jugs or bottles without putting a lid on them. Cover the tops with a few layers of cheesecloth, and hold them in place with an elastic band. Store the bottles or jars in a cool, dark place for three weeks to six months, depending on the level of tanginess you prefer in your apple cider vinegar. The longer the juice sits, the more acidic the vinegar will taste, while shorter times produce a taste more like juice and only mildly like vinegar. Keep in mind that some alcohol may develop during the process, so if you use your vinegar early in the fermentation cycle, it may actually taste more like apple cider wine than vinegar. Simply leave the apple juice/cider to ferment for a longer amount of time until the alcohol converts into acetic acid, which means it is now ready to use as vinegar.

If you purchased apple juice or apple cider, you can simply secure the cheesecloth over the top in place of the lid and store in a cool, dark place until it becomes vinegar.

You may notice a thick substance that forms on the top of the juice/vinegar. That's the "mother," as it is known — the collection of bacteria that form in the juice that are responsible for converting it to vinegar. You can save the mother to use as a starter culture for the next batch of apple cider or other type of vinegar if you'd like. Using an existing mother helps to slightly speed up the process of making vinegar. Once you're happy with the level of acidity, simply cap the bottles and store until you are ready to use. Enjoy!

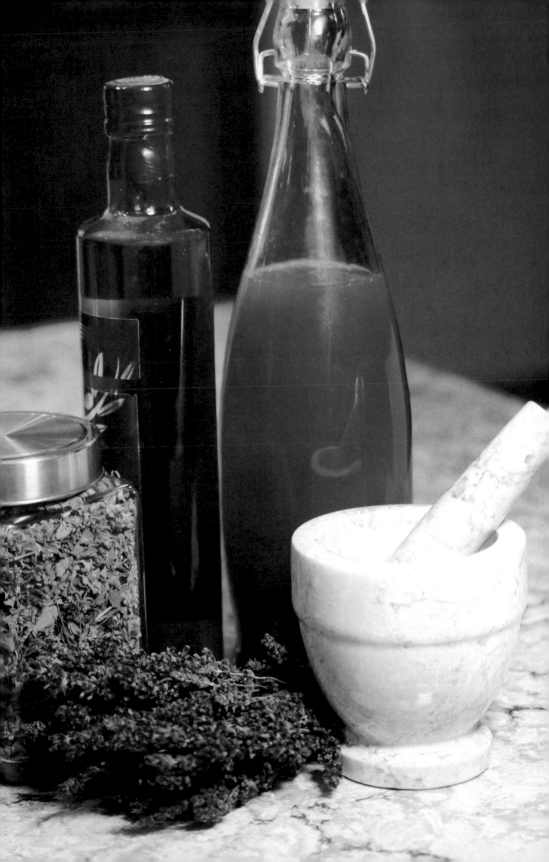

Seven Health Benefits of Apple Cider Vinegar and Other Natural Fruit Vinegars

Search the internet, and you will find countless claims about seemingly miraculous health benefits from consuming apple cider vinegar — but is it all true? I hit the research journals to separate fact from fiction and proven claims from the internet-sustained myths.

I discovered that although apple cider vinegar does indeed have many beneficial properties, most of the claims floating around in cyberspace are unfounded in research. So here are some of the evidence-based benefits of apple cider vinegar, which would also apply to apple vinegar (recipe on page 132):

1. Improves insulin sensitivity in people with diabetes. Several studies demonstrate vinegar's ability to improve insulin sensitivity and lower blood sugar responses when eaten as part of meals or taken before bedtime, which may offer help in treating diabetes. Research published in the medical journal *Annals of Nutrition and Metabolism* found that vinegar consumed with meals containing carbohydrates improved blood sugar levels by 20 percent.[1]

2. Regulates blood chemistry in people with diabetes. Improving insulin sensitivity isn't the only way apple cider vinegar appears to help diabetics; it has also been shown to help normalize other aspects of blood chemistry. Research showed that apple cider vinegar helped regulate blood chemistry, including cholesterol and triglyceride levels, of diabetic animals fed the vinegar as part of their regular diet for four weeks.[2]

3. Kills *E. Coli* on produce. The *Journal of Food Protection* assessed the effects of spraying various solutions on lettuce inoculated with *E. coli*.[3] Although the apple cider vinegar did not kill the *E. coli* completely, it did help to reduce the numbers of the bacteria linked with food poisoning while not affecting the taste of the lettuce or its crispness.

4. Regulates effects of dietary cholesterol. In a study published in the *Journal of Membrane Biology*, researchers studied the effects of a high cholesterol diet on animals fed apple cider vinegar versus animals that only ate the high cholesterol diet.[4] They found that the apple cider vinegar exerted a protective effect on the liver and kidneys, among other protective benefits. Considering that the liver is involved in over five hundred different functions — including neutralizing harsh chemicals, balancing hormones, and reducing the degenerative effects of cholesterol and the kidneys help to regulate blood pressure — it is a good idea to support them with healthy food choices.

5. Aids weight loss. While there are conflicting studies about apple cider vinegar's effects on obesity and weight loss, according to research in the *European Journal of Clinical Nutrition*, apple cider vinegar can help reduce the number of calories eaten at a meal by between 200 and 275 by making us feel full.[5] Additional study results published in the journal

Bioscience, Biotechnology, and Biochemistry also showed that vinegar helped obese individuals achieve weight loss.[6]

6. Helps fight heart disease. Apple cider vinegar contains the nutrient chlorogenic acid, which, according to a study published in the journal *Biochemical Pharmacology*, helps prevent LDL cholesterol, also known as the "bad cholesterol," from oxidizing, which is an important step in the progression of heart disease.[7]

7. Reduces bacteria in oral infections. A study published in the journal *Oral Surgery, Oral Medicine, Oral Pathology, Oral Radiology and Endodontics* found that apple cider vinegar demonstrated antibacterial activity against *E. faecalis* bacteria, which are linked to infection in root canals and elsewhere in the body.[8]

Are There Anticancer Effects?

There is a lot of internet hype about apple cider vinegar's alleged anticancer effects, but the research doesn't really support it. While some studies showed anticancer effects from rice vinegar and sugar cane vinegar in laboratory settings, there is little research supporting the claim that apple cider vinegar has any anticancer properties.[9] So it may prevent cancer; it may not — we'll have to wait for the research to find out.

How to Benefit

Keep in mind that you should never drink apple cider vinegar undiluted. The vinegar is an acid that can burn the delicate mucus membranes of the digestive tract, so always use it diluted in water or juice or mixed with oil in a salad dressing. Choose an unfiltered, unpasteurized apple cider vinegar with the "mother" left intact (the collection of beneficial microbes that convert apple cider into apple cider vinegar), or better yet, make the Crabapple Vinegar or Apple Vinegar recipes on pages 129 and 132. That way you'll know for sure that it contains live cultures and has not been bastardized with unnatural ingredients or pasteurization.

Pineapple Vinegar

Imagine having your pineapple (in the form of vinegar) and eating it too. That's completely possible when you remove the skins and core from a pineapple, eat the fleshy fruit, and reserve the scraps to make pineapple vinegar. Because pineapples can contain many pesticides and other unwanted ingredients, I recommend using an organic pineapple for your vinegar. You should also wash the whole pineapple prior to cutting it so as to remove any mold or harmful bacteria that may have found their way onto the surface of the pineapple. After tasting this delightful pineapple vinegar, you'll never look at fruit scraps the same way again.

Makes about ½ to 1 quart/liter

½ cup coconut sugar
1 quart filtered water
1 medium pineapple

In a pitcher or large measuring cup, mix together the sugar and water, stirring if necessary to encourage the sugar to dissolve.

Remove the skin and core from the pineapple. Set the meat of the fruit aside for another use. Coarsely chop the skins and core. Place the pineapple scraps in a 1- to 2-quart jar or crock, leaving about 1 to 2 inches at the top of the jar.

Pour the sugar-water solution over the pineapple skins and core, leaving about ¾ inch at the top of the jar. The pieces will float to the top, and some won't be submerged, but that's okay.

Cover the opening with a few layers of clean cheesecloth, and attach an elastic band around the mouth of the jar or crock to hold the cheesecloth in place.

Every day, remove the cheesecloth, and stir to cover the pineapple pieces with the sugar-water solution. You *must* do this every day to ensure that the pineapple pieces don't go moldy during the fermentation process. After two weeks, strain off the pineapple pieces, reserving the liquid; you can add the pineapple to your compost. Pour the liquid into a bottle, and seal with a tight-fitting lid or cork. The vinegar keeps for approximately one year.

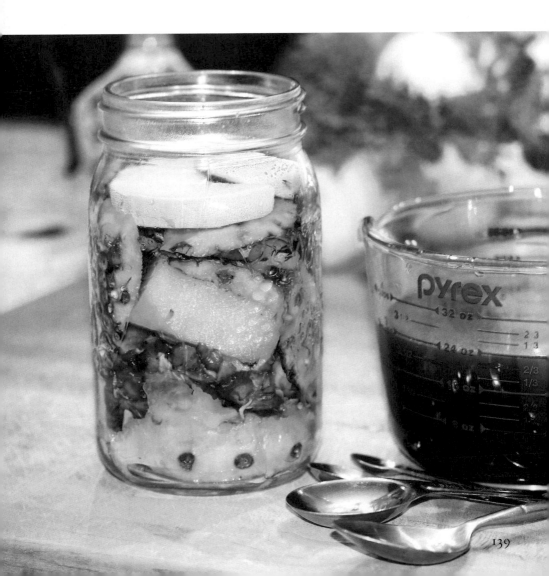

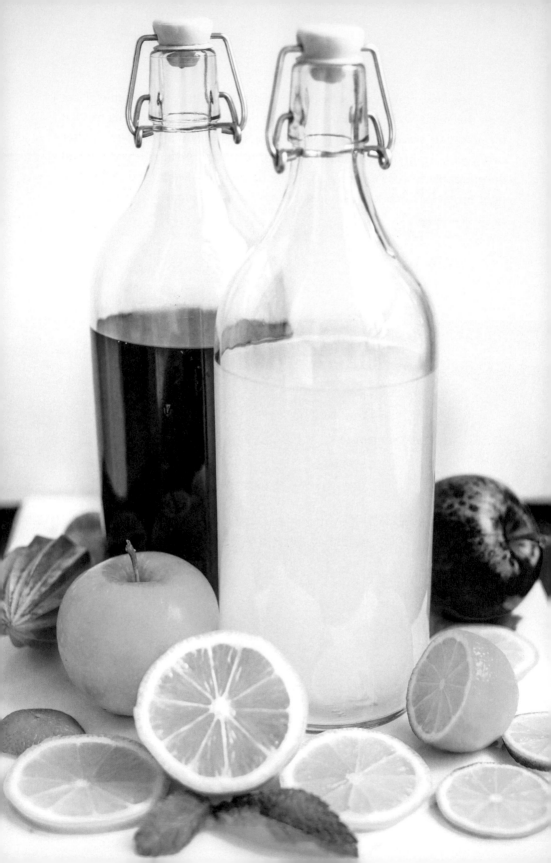

CHAPTER SIX

CULTURED BEVERAGES
Vegan Kefir, Kombucha, and More

In addition to lacto-fermented vegetables and cultured plant-based cheeses, you can also make many delightful fermented beverages full of healing probiotics. Don't let their lack of familiarity scare you off — they are actually simple to make. Once you've tried your first batch, you'll be hooked. In this chapter I'll explain how to make kefir and kombucha, and I'll even share a recipe that demonstrates how to use leftover sauerkraut or pickle brine as a starter culture for beverages.

In this chapter you'll discover the following recipes:

- Vegan Kefir
- Black Tea Kombucha
- African Red Tea Kombucha
- Cultured Nonalcoholic Bloody Mary

Kefir: Three Times Healthier Than Yogurt

While most people know about yogurt and its many health benefits, few people realize that there is a better bacterial booster in town. Kefir (pronounced *ke-FEER*) is similar to a drinkable form of yogurt, but it is so much healthier. It has a tart, tangy, slightly sour taste with a slight effervescence.

Kefir comes from the Turkish word *keif*, which means "good feeling," probably because it offers so many health benefits — and many people report feeling good when they drink it regularly. Originally created in the Caucasus Mountains in Eastern Europe, it has a slightly thinner consistency than yogurt. It is made with kefir grains, which aren't actually grains and contain no gluten at all but a combination of various bacteria and yeasts. Some commercial kefir products are made with powdered kefir starter, which isn't truly authentic. As with yogurt, many commercial, bottled kefir products are frequently heavily sweetened and flavored, so be sure to read the labels if you're buying premade kefir. Or, better yet, make your own.

There are many reasons to consider adding kefir to your diet:

- It offers a bigger beneficial bacterial boost than yogurt, typically offering three times as many probiotics as yogurt. Additionally, it contains ten to twenty different strains of probiotics, whereas yogurt usually contains only two or three.
- It gives you a B-vitamin and energy boost. Kefir naturally contains several B-complex vitamins, including thiamine, folic acid, riboflavin, and biotin. B-complex vitamins are known as the energy vitamins because they are needed for energy production in the body. And even though many people continue to believe the myth that vitamin B12 is only found in meat, kefir is actually a good source of this valuable and essential nutrient.
- It improves dairy digestion. Many people who have trouble digesting dairy products are able to digest kefir because of its ability to improve the dairy's digestibility by breaking down some of the hard-to-digest proteins. During the fermentation process probiotics consume the milk sugars (lactose) as food. However, you don't need to drink dairy kefir to benefit from this delicious superfood; kefir can also be made with nondairy beverages such as coconut milk, almond milk, or rice milk, as well as juices. You'll find my recipe for Vegan Kefir on page 144.
- It regulates blood sugar and cholesterol. According to research published in the medical journal *Biofactors*, kefir has been shown

to reduce cholesterol levels, lower blood sugar, and prevent blood sugar spikes, making it a good choice in the prevention or treatment of heart disease.[1]

- It lowers blood glucose levels, a factor in diabetes, so it may help people with diabetes better manage their disease.[2]

- Regular kefir consumption has also been shown to prevent blood pressure spikes in animals.[3] These effects would likely be found in humans as well.

- Kefir has shown potential for preventing or treating fatty liver disease, a common ailment in those who have difficulty losing weight as well as in many people with diabetes.

- Cutting-edge research has shown that the probiotics found in some kefir products may help in the treatment of cancer. One type of probiotic, *Lactobacillus kefiri P-IF*, was shown to help destroy human leukemia cells — even when multiple cancer drugs were unable to induce the cancer cell–killing process. The scientists concluded that the novel kefir bacteria "may act as a potential therapy for the treatment of multidrug-resistant leukemia."[4]

If you are purchasing kefir products, beware of products with added flavors and sugars. To ensure that your kefir is free from unhealthy added ingredients, try creating your own. What you make at home will be far superior to most of the bottled varieties. Kefir is easy to make on an ongoing basis, so you can keep a regular supply to boost your health. It takes only a couple of minutes to add the kefir grains (which are not actually grain products at all) to the milk, dairy-free milk, or juice you're using, then twenty-four to forty-eight hours to ferment. Because probiotic cultures tend to dwindle over time during storage, making your own is also a good way to ensure the integrity of the probiotic cultures in your kefir. I recommend using kefir grains over starter powder for a more authentic kefir that is full of live cultures.

On page 144 you'll find step-by-step instructions on how to make kefir. You'll only need a sterilized glass jar, a mesh (not metal) sieve, kefir grains, and milk, nondairy milk, juice, or some other beverage. You can drink kefir on its own, stir in vanilla or cocoa for a flavored beverage, add it to your breakfast cereal, or add fruit and whip it into a delicious smoothie.

Vegan Kefir

Traditionally kefir is made using cow's milk, but you can also make kefir with plant-based milks. Here's a simple recipe for making your own kefir from cashew milk, but feel free to try other types of milk as well, such as almond, sunflower seed, or coconut. The sweetener feeds the kefir microbes, so there will be minimal sugar left in the final product. You'll notice that the grains will grow in number over time. You only need about one tablespoon of kefir grains to keep your kefir going, so you can remove the extras and either eat them, give them to friends, or put them in the compost.

Makes about 1 quart/liter

1 quart (or liter) filtered water
½ cup raw, unsalted cashews
1 teaspoon coconut sugar, pure maple syrup, or agave nectar
1 tablespoon kefir grains
Mandarin sections for garnish (optional)

In a blender, blend together the water, cashews, and coconut sugar (or maple syrup or agave nectar) until it is smooth and creamy. Pour the cashew milk into a 1½- to 2-quart glass jar, making sure that it is less than ⅔ full. Add the kefir grains, stir, and place the cap on the jar.

Leave the jar at room temperature for twenty-four to forty-eight hours, gently agitating it periodically. The cashew milk will become somewhat bubbly, then it will begin to coagulate and separate; simply shake it to remix the kefir, or scoop out the thicker curds and use them as you would use soft cheese or sour cream. Refrigerate for up to one week. When ready to serve the kefir, pour it into a glass and garnish the rim of the glass with mandarin sections, if desired.

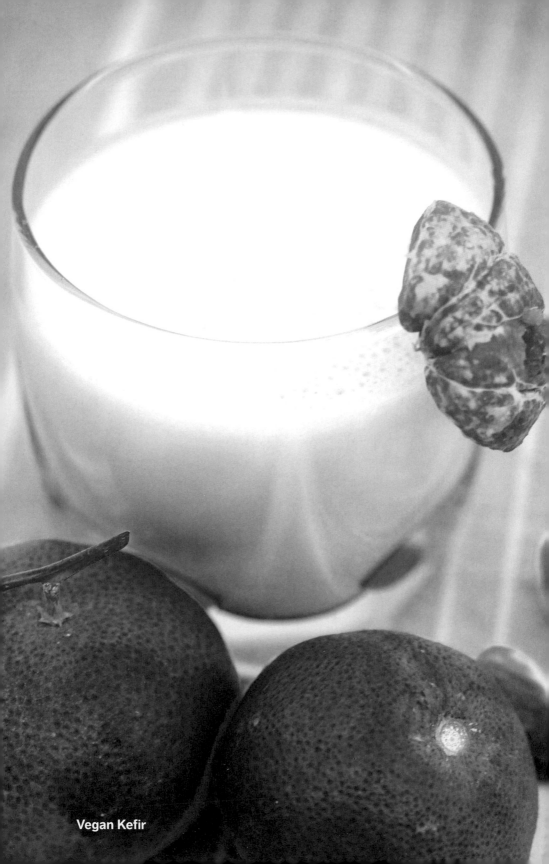

Vegan Kefir

Kombucha: The Natural Soda That Promotes Vitality

Kombucha (pronounced *kom-BOO-shuh* — notice the *sh* sound) is a beverage believed to have been first developed in Russia more than two millennia ago. An odd-looking bacteria-and-yeast combination forms the signature kombucha culture, which actually looks like a floating mat on the surface of the tea or juice from which kombucha — the beverage — is made.

While there hasn't been a lot of research conducted on the health benefits of kombucha, there is a large body of anecdotal evidence, some of which has been compiled into whole books on the drink. Recently the Laboratory of Industrial Microbiology and Food Biotechnology at the University of Latvia assessed existing research on the health benefits of kombucha tea and found that it has four main healing properties: first, it improves detoxification; second, it has antioxidant properties that can counter the effects of harmful free radicals in the body; third, it has energizing effects; and fourth, it improves immunity against some diseases. According to their research, consuming kombucha could potentially help us prevent a broad spectrum of metabolic and infectious disorders.[5]

Because so many people today live with diabetes, any natural food that demonstrates effectiveness in improving diabetic symptoms and reducing associated health conditions should be considered a valuable option for people with diabetes. In a preliminary study published in *Food and Chemical Toxicology*, researchers at the Department of Life Sciences and Biotechnology at Jadavpur University in India studied the antioxidant effects of fermented black tea kombucha compared to the effects of black tea on diabetic animals. Their results showed the "significant anti-diabetic potential" of kombucha. While the black tea was helpful, the researchers believe the higher levels of antioxidants in the kombucha could be responsible for its superior results.[6]

Both bacteria and yeasts ferment the sweetened tea, including *Gluconacetobacter*, which laboratory analysis has found to be the dominant bacteria present in kombucha tea (sometimes greater than 85 percent of the bacteria), *Lactobacilli* (up to 30 percent of the bacteria), and trace amounts of *Acetobacter* (less than 2 percent). The yeast populations are dominated by Zygosaccharomyces, which comprises more than 95 percent of the yeast in the fermented beverage.[7]

In a study conducted at the College of Engineering at China Agricultural University in Beijing and published in the *Journal of the Science of Food and Agriculture*, researchers explored the liver-protective properties of kombucha to determine which microorganism(s) and chemical constituents might be responsible for these protective effects observed from kombucha. In this study, researchers assessed kombucha's ability to protect the animals against liver injury resulting from acetaminophen (Tylenol is one of the main brand names of acetaminophen). They attributed the liver-protecting effects to a chemical compound made by *Gluconacetobacter sp. A4* bacteria found in kombucha tea.[8]

Furthermore, new research published in the journal *Current Microbiology* found that kombucha showed significant potency against numerous illness-causing bacteria, including *E. coli* and *Salmonella*, both of which are linked to food poisoning.[9]

There are many excellent store-bought varieties of kombucha, but I encourage you to make your own. It is a simple process, as you'll soon discover. And you don't need to make a new batch every time; rather, you can just keep adding tea to the batch you have, and it will ferment so you can have kombucha always on hand.

Grow Your Own Kombucha Starter

I discovered a simple trick to getting a kombucha starter culture, known as *scoby*. It's as simple as buying an unflavored bottle of kombucha from your local health-food or grocery store. Empty the contents into a small glass or ceramic bowl. Secure a few layers of cheesecloth or a layer of muslin to the top with a rubber band. Let it sit in an undisturbed spot in your kitchen for two weeks. You should see a rubbery mass floating on top. Congratulations! You just grew your own scoby that you can now use to make your own batch of kombucha. (*Note:* Make sure the kombucha beverage you purchase has not been pasteurized and contains live cultures.) You may notice a small amount of sediment in the bottom of the bottle — that's the beginning of a new scoby forming!

Black Tea Kombucha

Few people would claim soda is healthy, contrary to what manufacturers of the sugary stuff would say. In fact, with a whopping 39 grams of sugar per can of cola, soda is completely unhealthy. But there is one type of soda that is naturally brewed and lightly carbonated and is made by fermenting tea. Unlike the sugar-, color-, and preservative-laden canned drinks, kombucha is packed with health-building microbes and is easier to make than you might think. Here are my step-by-step instructions for making your own kombucha at home. And don't worry about the sugar content: most of the sugar is consumed by the beneficial bacteria during the fermentation process.

Note: Avoid drinking kombucha if you have an ulcer, as the acetic acid that naturally forms during the fermentation process can irritate ulcers.

Makes about 3½ quarts/liters

4 quarts (or liters) filtered water
1 cup unrefined sugar
4 black tea bags or 4 heaping teaspoons loose-leaf tea
1 kombucha starter culture (also called the "mother"; see "Grow Your Own Kombucha
  Starter" on page 147, or find one in almost any health food store or get one from
  someone in your community who makes his or her own kombucha)

In a large stainless-steel pot, bring the water to a boil, add the sugar, and stir until the sugar is fully dissolved. Add the black tea bags or loose tea, and boil for an additional 10 minutes to kill off any unwanted microbes that may be present on the tea bags. Turn off the heat, and allow the tea to steep for 15 minutes; remove the tea bags. (If using loose leaf tea, simply use a sieve when pouring the cool tea into the kombucha crock; compost the used tea leaves.)

Allow the tea to cool to room temperature or slightly lukewarm temperature; it should be no warmer than about 70°F or 21°C to ensure that the kombucha culture is not damaged. Pour the steeped tea into a large ceramic crock or wide-mouthed glass water jug, such as those used to make iced tea. (I use a crock with a spigot on the side, but any inexpensive glass water jug with a spigot works. Make sure the crock or jug is thoroughly cleaned prior to use.)

Add to the tea the kombucha starter culture along with any tea it came with. Cover the top of the crock or jug with a piece of clean linen or cotton (avoid using cheesecloth, as it is too porous), and attach an elastic band around the rim to hold the cloth in place; alternatively, you can use tape around the edge to hold the cloth in place and ensure that the cloth doesn't fall into the crock or jug.

Place the crock or jug someplace quiet with air ventilation, in a warm but not sunlit area, where it will not be disturbed. The ideal fermentation temperature range is 73 to 82°F, or 23 to 28°C. Once you've located a spot for it, do not move the crock or jug while the kombucha is fermenting, as it may interfere with the culturing process.

Wait about five to six days to harvest your kombucha. First, check the taste: If it is sweeter than you'd like, allow it to ferment another day or two. If it has a vinegary taste, you may need to bottle future batches after fermenting a shorter period of time; it is still fine to drink, but you may need to dilute it with water when you drink it to avoid irritating your throat or stomach.

Pour all but approximately 2 cups of your fermented kombucha into a glass jar, a container with a lid, or multiple single-serving resealable glass jars (old-fashioned soda pop bottles with the flip-top lid work well), cover, and store it in the refrigerator. To increase its fizziness, add a pinch of sugar, and wait another day or two to drink it. If you keep it longer than a week, you may need to loosen the lid in the fridge to allow gases to escape and prevent the glass from breaking due to excess pressure that may occur over longer periods of time. It will keep in the fridge for up to a year, but you'll want to let the gases escape by opening the lid every week or two, otherwise you could have an explosion in your kitchen. Just ask my friend Alanah, who, along with a few of her family members, spent an hour cleaning her kitchen after her kombucha exploded.

That's it. You made your first batch of healthy soda. Enjoy!

African Red Tea Kombucha

I love the natural vanilla-like flavor of rooibos (pronounced *ROY-bus*) tea, which is also sometimes called African red tea because the plant originates in parts of Africa. It has a naturally sweet flavor and delightful taste when fermented using a kombucha scoby culture. This delicious and slightly effervescent cultured beverage is easy to make.

Makes about 3½ quarts/liters

4 quarts filtered water
1 cup coconut sugar
4 teaspoons rooibos loose-leaf tea or 4 rooibos tea bags
1 kombucha starter culture (also called the "mother"; see "Grow Your Own Kombucha
   Starter" on page 147, or find one in almost any health food store or get one from
   someone in your community who makes his or her own kombucha)

In a large stainless-steel pot, bring the water to a boil, add the sugar, and stir until the sugar is fully dissolved. Add the rooibos tea bags or loose tea, and boil for an additional 10 minutes to kill off any unwanted microbes that may be present on the tea bags. Turn off the heat, and allow the tea to steep for 15 minutes; remove the tea bags.

Let the tea cool to room temperature or slightly lukewarm temperature; it should be no warmer than about 70°F or 21°C to ensure that the kombucha culture is not damaged. Pour the steeped tea into a large ceramic crock or wide-mouthed glass water jug, through a fine-mesh sieve in order to remove any loose-leaf tea (if using).

Add to the tea the kombucha starter culture along with any tea it came with. Cover the top of the crock or jug with a piece of clean linen or cotton (avoid using cheesecloth, as it is too porous), and attach an elastic band around the rim to hold the cloth in place; alternatively, you can use tape around the edge to hold the cloth in place and ensure that the cloth doesn't fall into the crock or jug.

Place the crock or jug someplace quiet with air ventilation, in a warm but not sunlit area, where it will not be disturbed. The ideal fermentation temperature range is 73 to 82°F, or 23 to 28°C. Once you've located a spot for it, do not move the crock or jug while the kombucha is fermenting, as it may interfere with the culturing process.

Wait about five to six days to harvest your kombucha. First, check the taste: If it is sweeter than you'd like, allow it to ferment another day or two. If it has a vinegary taste, you may need to bottle future batches after a shorter period of time; it is still fine to drink, but you may need to dilute it with water when you drink it to avoid irritating your throat or stomach.

Pour all but approximately 2 cups of your fermented kombucha into a glass jar or container with a lid, or multiple single-serving resealable glass jars (old-fashioned soda pop bottles with the flip-top lid work well), cover, and store it in the refrigerator. To increase its fizziness, add a pinch of sugar, and wait another a day or two to drink it. If you keep it longer than a week, you may need to loosen the lid in the fridge to allow gases to escape and prevent the glass from breaking due to excess pressure that may occur over longer periods of time. It will store for up to one year in the fridge, but you'll need to release the gases every week or two by opening the lids or caps on the bottles.

Note: Avoid drinking kombucha if you have an ulcer, as the acetic acid that naturally forms during the fermentation process can irritate ulcers.

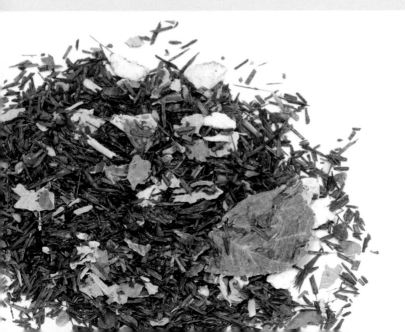

Cultured Nonalcoholic Bloody Mary

I created this recipe as a way to use leftover sauerkraut or pickle brine after all the sauerkraut and pickles have been eaten. The brine is full of nutrients and probiotics, making it a shame to just throw out. So I thought, "Why not use it as a starter culture for a vegetable cocktail?" And that's how my cultured Bloody Mary came about. This delicious juice increases your vegetable (well, technically, fruit, as tomatoes and limes are fruit) intake while also nourishing your body with plentiful amounts of beneficial microbes. I used kimchi brine from the White Kimchi recipe on page 122, but feel free to use a different kind if you prefer. Of course, feel free to add a splash of vodka if you'd like a probiotic-rich cocktail.

Makes about 2 cups

4 medium tomatoes
Juice from ½ lime
⅓ cup brine from kimchi, sauerkraut, or pickles
Dash unrefined sea salt
Dash pepper
1 stalk celery (optional, for garnish)

In a blender, combine all the ingredients except the celery, and blend until it is smooth. Pour the mixture into a covered glass dish, and allow it to ferment for two to twelve hours, depending on your preference; longer fermentation times result in a tangier drink. (It is not necessary to ferment the juice if you'd rather not, since you're using brine from previously fermented kimchi, sauerkraut, or pickles.) Garnish with celery if desired, and serve immediately. Store any leftovers in a jar in the fridge for up to three days.

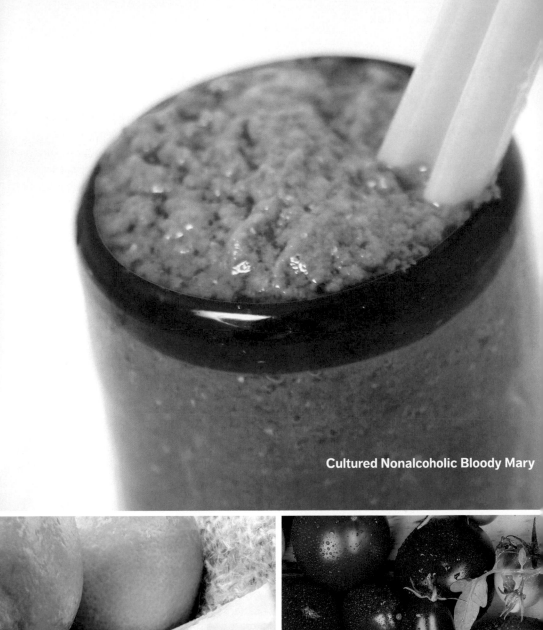

Cultured Nonalcoholic Bloody Mary

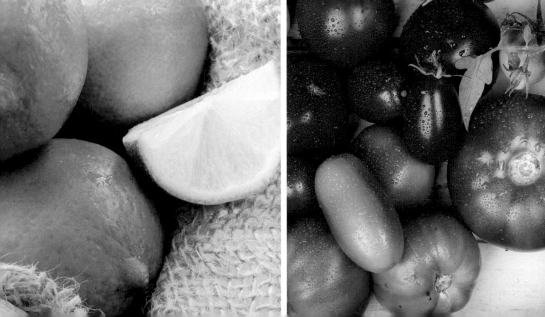

How to Make Kombucha on an Ongoing Basis

You can keep a crock or jar of kombucha perpetually brewing on your countertop by following the instructions for a single batch and then making some minor modifications.

First, make your initial batch of kombucha according to the directions on page 148. On day five or six, boil a new pot of tea according to the instructions, and let cool. Leaving only the scoby (the starter culture) and a cup or two of the tea in the kombucha crock, bottle the kombucha that is already made, and refrigerate it in bottles. (Remember to drink these within a week or two, or to periodically open the bottles to let the gases out. Otherwise the bottles can explode from built-up pressure.) When your new batch of tea has sufficiently cooled, pour it into the kombucha crock. Switching between types of tea (green, black, rooibos, or other tea) should be no problem as long as the cup or two of the old batch has a flavor profile that complements the new one. You can still use the same scoby. I regularly make black tea kombucha and then switch it to green tea or rooibos. Simply mark on the calendar five or six days from the start date of your kombucha, bottle this batch, and then brew a new one.

CHAPTER SEVEN

RECIPES FOR USING YOUR CULTURED CREATIONS

By now you've learned how to make many health-building and delicious cultured foods, from yogurt and sauerkraut to fruit cultures and vegan cheeses. In this chapter you will learn how to make many other exciting fermented creations, including fermented ice cream and cheesecake. You'll also learn how to use other cultured creations you made earlier in this book, as well as discover twenty-five ways to incorporate fermented foods into your daily diet. The recipes include:

- Tzatziki (Greek-Style Yogurt Cucumber Dip)
- Creamy French Onion Dip
- Mixed Green Salad with Grilled Peaches and Chèvrew
- Coconut Cream Cheese Icing
- Cardamom Pear Crêpes with Macadamia Cream Cheese
- Gingerbread Cookie Ice Cream Sandwiches
- Cultured Vanilla Ice Cream
- Pumpkin Pie Ice Cream
- Black Cherry Ice Cream
- Orange Creamsicle Cheesecake

- Dairy-Free Pomegranate Cheesecake
- Blackberry Cheesecake

For the ice cream recipes you may wish to invest in an ice cream machine, as it can make light work of homemade ice cream. Plus, once you've tasted homemade dairy-free ice cream, you'll probably never want to go back to the unhealthy store-bought varieties. What's more, ice cream makers have really come down in price, with some as low as $30. But even if you don't have an ice cream machine, you can still make the ice cream recipes in this book: simply follow the instructions in the recipes, and then pour the ice cream mixture into a stainless-steel bowl and gently place it in the freezer. Every thirty to forty-five minutes remove the bowl from the freezer, and whisk the contents until fairly smooth. Return to the freezer and repeat this process until the mixture reaches the consistency of ice cream.

Twenty-Five Ways to Get More Fermented Foods into Your Diet

If you're like many people, outside of yogurt with fruit or sauerkraut on your favorite hot dog or sausage, you may not know how to get more fermented foods into your daily diet. While there are countless possibilities, here are twenty-five of my favorite ways to eat more fermented foods:

Using Yogurt or Kefir

1. Smoothies. Blend some yogurt or kefir with a handful or two of fruit for a delicious smoothie.
2. Frozen yogurt. After making a fruit smoothie with yogurt or kefir, pour it into popsicle molds and freeze for a frozen yogurt treat.
3. Yogurt cheese. Pour yogurt into a cheesecloth-lined sieve, and let it sit for at least a few hours for a soft yogurt cheese — simply add your favorite herbs for an unbeatable fresh cheese. (Like all the yogurt-based suggestions, these approaches work for vegan yogurt as well.)
4. Yogurt salad dressing. Blend some yogurt with lemon juice or vinegar, along with some herbs and sea salt, for a creamy salad dressing.
5. Save yogurt to make more. Save a few tablespoons of yogurt or the whey from yogurt making to serve as the starter culture for your

next batch. Doing this will not only save you money, but you'll also be able to eat more yogurt.

6. Breakfast cereal. Add a dollop or two of yogurt or kefir to your favorite breakfast cereal or oatmeal in place of milk.

Using Sauerkraut, Pickled Vegetables, or Kimchi

7. Over brown rice or quinoa for a quick meal. Simply adding sauerkraut, kimchi, pickled vegetables, or other fermented vegetables to cooked grains makes a quick, nutritious, and delicious meal.

8. Over salad. I threw some sauerkraut on top of a homemade Caesar salad, and it was delicious. You can add fermented veggies to almost any salad for a quick probiotic boost.

9. On noodles. Tossing brown rice or other whole grain noodles with kimchi or pickled veggies makes mealtime a cinch.

10. Sandwiches. Adding pickled turnips, fermented onions, cultured radishes, kimchi, or sauerkraut to your favorite sandwich gives it a flavor and nutritional boost.

11. and 12. On burgers and hot dogs. This one is self-explanatory.

13. Lettuce cups. Place freshly grated vegetables, bean sprouts, and fermented veggies or kimchi in a large leaf of lettuce, and wrap it up for a simple snack or meal.

14. Salad rolls. Soak rice paper wraps in hot water, pat dry, and wrap them around fermented and fresh veggies.

15. Tacos. Top your favorite tacos with fermented vegetables such as carrots or onions for a flavor boost. Keep Taco Pickles (page 118) in your fridge, and you'll have the perfect accompaniment for your next taco night.

16. Salad dressing. Blend sauerkraut or kimchi with two parts oil and one part vinegar for a quick and easy salad dressing. You can also save the sauerkraut juice and use it in place of vinegar and salt in your next salad dressing.

17. Condiments. Add pickled vegetables or kimchi as a condiment to almost any meal.

18. Guacamole. I often mix Salvadoran Salsa (page 106) with mashed avocado for a simple and amazingly delicious chunky guacamole in minutes.

19. Salsa and chips. Mix fresh salsa ingredients like chopped tomatoes, onion, garlic, lemon juice, and minced chilis with the contents of one probiotic capsule or one-quarter teaspoon of probiotic powder, and let sit for at least a few hours, preferably overnight. Then serve your fermented salsa with chips for a great snack.

20. Hummus. Blend sauerkraut (or sauerkraut juice) and chickpeas with a little extra-virgin olive oil, lemon, and tahini (sesame butter) for a quick and probiotic-rich hummus. The sauerkraut and sauerkraut juice add flavor and replace salt in this recipe.

Using Other Fermented Foods

21. Fermented juice. Empty the contents of a probiotic capsule, or sprinkle one-quarter teaspoon of probiotic powder, into your favorite fruit or vegetable juice, cover, and leave at room temperature overnight or for twenty-four hours. Not only will you get the probiotics from the capsule, but the beneficial microbes will also proliferate and actually reduce the amount of natural sugars present in the juice. I often do this before bed and enjoy probiotic-rich juice with breakfast in the morning.

22. Choose kombucha over soda. Skip the sugar-laden soft drink, and instead enjoy a naturally sparkling kombucha.

23. Cultured cream. Soak raw, unsalted nuts like cashews, pine nuts, or macadamias in enough water to cover along with the contents of one probiotic capsule or one-quarter teaspoon probiotic powder. Let sit for eight hours or overnight, then blend. Dollop over fruit in place of cream. Or, for a thick vegan sour cream, use only as much of the soak water as needed to attain the desired thickness, and extend the culturing time to twenty-four hours; you can also add some lemon juice to increase the tart taste.

24. Vegan cheese. Follow the instructions for number 23, cultured cream, but use only enough water to cover the nuts, then allow them to ferment with the probiotic powder for at least twenty-four hours or, for a sharper cheese flavor, up to forty-eight hours. Any longer

than that and you may start to develop unwanted mold. Then blend until smooth and creamy for a quick and probiotic-rich soft cheese. 25. Vegan pudding or cheesecake. Follow the instructions for number 24, vegan cheese, but skip the salt and add some fruit and sweetener (if you wish), along with a couple of tablespoons of a thickening agent like ground chia or flax seeds. For a cheesecake, crumble some graham crackers or cookies with a small amount of coconut oil, and press into a small cheesecake mold. Then pour the fruit-cashew mixture over the crust, refrigerate until firm, et voilà! Enjoy this simple, raw, probiotic-rich pudding or cheesecake. For a superb cultured cheesecake, be sure to try my recipe for Orange Creamsicle Cheesecake on page 178.

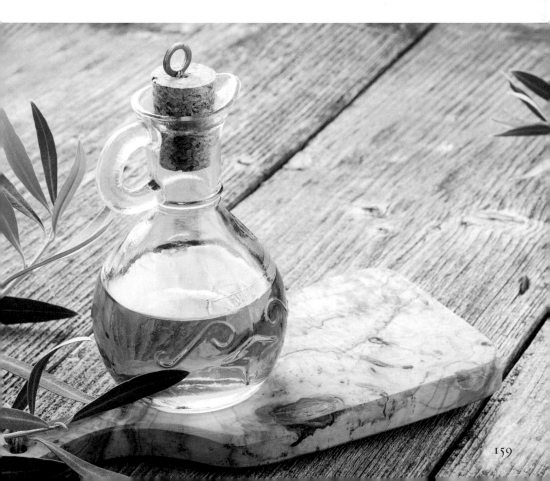

Tzatziki (Greek-Style Yogurt Cucumber Dip)

This is my dairy-free take on one of my favorite foods, tzatziki. Tzatziki is a traditional Greek dip made from thick, Greek-style yogurt with grated onions, garlic, cucumbers, and lemon juice. This version is so creamy and delicious that you'll quickly forget there is no dairy in it. Not only does the taste measure up to the more commonly known dairy version, but it also contains even more probiotics than the original. Your taste buds *and* your gut will thank you! Serve tzatziki with cooked or raw vegetables; over your favorite veggie burgers, sausages, or meatballs; or on a sandwich or in a wrap with your favorite fixings. You can also toss romaine lettuce or baby spinach greens with tzatziki in place of salad dressing for a savory probiotic-rich lunch or dinner.

Makes about 1½ to 2 cups

1 cup raw, unsalted cashews
½ cup filtered water
1 probiotic capsule or ¼ teaspoon probiotic powder
Juice from 1 lemon
1 garlic clove, minced
2 tablespoons minced onion
1 teaspoon unrefined sea salt
One 3-inch piece of a medium cucumber (or about ½ cup grated, drained, and packed
    cucumber), plus additional cucumber slices and/or slivers, for garnish (optional)

In a small to medium glass bowl, combine the cashews and water. Empty the contents of the probiotic capsule (discarding the empty capsule shell) or probiotic powder into the cashew mixture, and stir to combine. Cover and set aside for twenty-four hours. Alternatively, you can use 1½ cups of the World's Easiest Yogurt (page 44).

In a blender, combine the cashew mixture with the lemon juice, garlic, onion, and salt, and blend until smooth and creamy; return the mixture to the bowl. Grate the cucumber, add it to the cashew mixture, and stir until combined. Store, covered, in the refrigerator for up to three days. When ready to serve, garnish with cucumber slices and/or slivers, if desired.

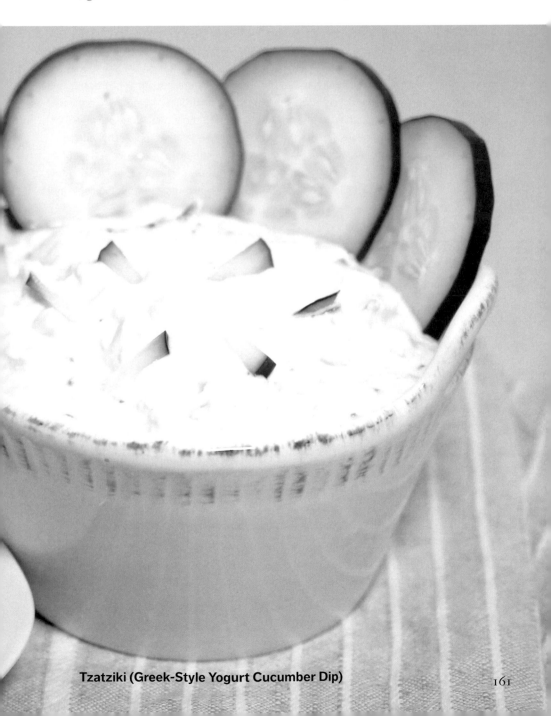

Tzatziki (Greek-Style Yogurt Cucumber Dip)

Creamy French Onion Dip

When I was a teenager I babysat almost every evening and weekend for two families. Without knowing my snack preferences, both sets of parents regularly left chips and French onion dip for me to snack on, which, admittedly, I loved. As the years passed, I gave up these less-than-healthy snacks in favor of healthier options, but one day many years later I suddenly had a craving for this snack and went to work to make a healthier and fermented version of it. The result: French Onion Dip! But unlike the store-bought versions, this one has no dairy, no hydrogenated oils or preservatives, and no artificial flavors. This is the real deal, but it tastes so good that no one will know you fed them a much healthier option. Curtis and I keep a bowl of this dip on hand to enjoy with vegetable crudités, baked veggie chips, or whole-grain crackers. You'll probably eat it for the taste alone, but you can feel great about your decision, knowing it is packed with healthy probiotics too. Allowing this dip to refrigerate for at least a few hours after preparation allows the flavors to mingle and further improves flavor.

Makes about 2½ cups

2 cups raw, unsalted cashews
1½ cups filtered water
2 probiotic capsules or ½ teaspoon probiotic powder
Juice from ½ lemon
2 tablespoons minced green onion
2 tablespoons minced fresh parsley
About 1 teaspoon unrefined sea salt, or to taste
Chives or spring onions for garnish (optional)

In a small to medium glass bowl, combine the cashews and water. Empty the contents of the probiotic capsules (discarding the empty capsule shells) or probiotic powder into the cashews, and stir to mix. Cover and allow the mixture to culture for twenty-four to forty-eight hours. When ready to serve, garnish with chives or spring onions, if desired.

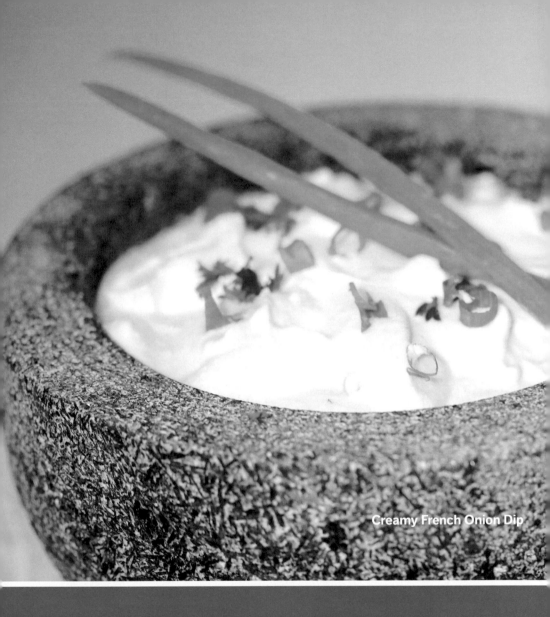

Creamy French Onion Dip

In a blender, pour the cashew mixture, and blend until smooth. Transfer to a medium bowl, add the lemon juice, and fold in the green onion and parsley until combined. Add salt to taste. Serve immediately or refrigerate for later use. This dip keeps in the refrigerator for about four days.

Mixed Green Salad with Grilled Peaches and Chèvrew

This gourmet salad has a beautiful blend of sweet and savory flavors, and the silky, creamy Chèvrew cheese is a textural sensation against the delicate greens. It is ideal in the summer months when fresh peaches are in season, but it's so good that you'll want to enjoy it year-round.

Serves 2 to 4

Salad

1 small package mesclun greens (mixed greens)
2 to 3 fresh peaches, pitted and halved
1 tablespoon extra-virgin olive oil
1-inch round Chèvrew (see page 70)

Dressing

¾ cup extra-virgin olive oil
⅓ cup apple cider vinegar
½ teaspoon unrefined sea salt
½ teaspoon dried basil
½ teaspoon dried thyme
1 teaspoon pure maple syrup or agave nectar

Preheat your barbecue to 300 to 350°F, or heat a cast-iron grill pan on your stovetop over low to medium heat.

Wash and dry the mesclun greens, and place in a large bowl; set aside.

Brush the peach halves with olive oil, and place flat side down on the barbecue or grill pan. Grill for about 3 minutes, or until peaches are soft but not mushy. Remove the peaches from the grill, turn off the heat, and set aside.

Cut the Chèvrew into discs, and set aside.

In a blender, combine all dressing ingredients, and blend until smooth. Pour your desired amount of dressing over the mixed greens, and toss the salad until it is well coated. Store any leftover dressing in a covered jar for up to one week.

Top the salad with the Chèvrew discs and grilled peach halves, and serve in large bowls or on plates.

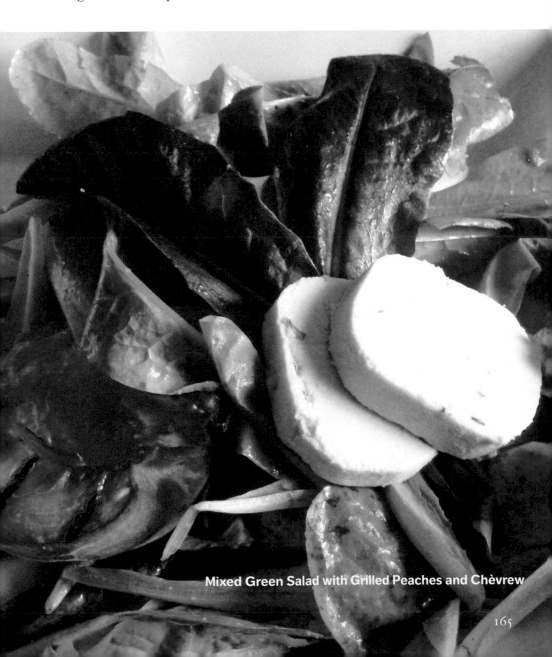

Mixed Green Salad with Grilled Peaches and Chèvrew

Coconut Cream Cheese Icing

You can use this icing recipe on all your favorite baked goods, from cupcakes to cakes and brownies. Not only is it a delicious dairy-free option, but it is also packed with health-building probiotics, so you can feel a lot less guilty about enjoying it.

One 13.5-ounce can coconut milk (use the regular version, not the "low-fat" or "light" options)
1 probiotic capsule or ¼ teaspoon probiotic powder
1 to 2 teaspoons pure maple syrup
1 teaspoon vanilla powder or pure vanilla extract
1 teaspoon lemon zest (optional)

Open the can of coconut milk. If the coconut cream and water have already separated, scoop off the thick cream into a small bowl. If it has not separated, in a small bowl simply mix both the coconut cream and coconut water together until smooth. Add the contents of the probiotic capsule (discarding the empty capsule shell) or probiotic powder, and mix together. Cover with a lid or cloth, and allow it to sit undisturbed for eight to ten hours in a warm setting (approximately 110 to 115°F or 43 to 46°C, but don't worry if it's not quite within that range).

After it has cultured, refrigerate for at least one to two hours. If the coconut cream and water have separated, scoop off the thickened coconut cream for use. (You can save the coconut water for other uses, such as smoothies, juices, or as a yogurt or cheese starter culture.) Add the maple syrup, vanilla powder or extract, and lemon zest if desired. Stir together until smooth. Use immediately as an icing for cakes, cupcakes, or other baked goods.

Lasts about one week, covered, in the fridge.

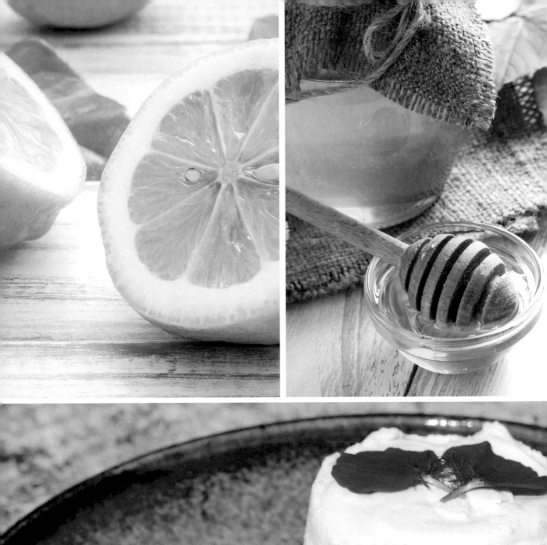

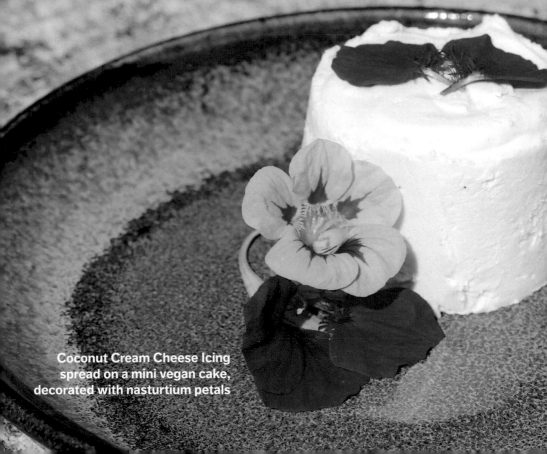

Coconut Cream Cheese Icing
spread on a mini vegan cake,
decorated with nasturtium petals

Cardamom Pear Crêpes ───────
with Macadamia Cream Cheese

One of my husband's friends, a kind farmer named Greg, gave us a box full of pears he grew on his farm. Inspired by his sweet gesture, I made this recipe for brunch. Curtis went back for seconds…and thirds…and fourths. I'd say it was a hit. Of course, if you eat eggs, feel free to replace the flaxseed-water mixture or Ener-G-water mixture with 2 eggs.

Makes 8 large crêpes

Crêpes

2 tablespoons olive oil, plus more for oiling frying pan
1½ cups all-purpose gluten-free flour (I use Bob's Red Mill xanthan-free flour)
1½ cups almond milk
2 tablespoons finely ground flaxseed whisked into 6 tablespoons water, or 3 teaspoons
    Ener-G Egg Replacer whisked into 4 tablespoons water
1 teaspoon baking soda
Pinch unrefined sea salt

Cardamom Pear Topping

4 medium pears, cored and sliced
Pinch ground cardamom
½ cup filtered water, divided
2 tablespoons organic cane sugar
1 tablespoon tapioca flour

Cream Cheese Topping

Macadamia Cream Cheese (see page 72)

For the crêpe batter, in a large bowl combine the 2 tablespoons oil, flour, almond milk, flaxseed-water mixture or Ener-G-water mixture, baking soda, and salt; whisk together.

In a large frying pan over medium heat, add enough oil to grease the entire bottom of the pan, and pour enough crêpe batter to thinly coat the pan. Cook for approximately 1 minute or until the bubbles disappear, and flip. Repeat with the remaining batter until the batter is all used up.

For the topping, in a medium frying pan over low to medium heat, add the pears, cardamom, and ¼ cup of the water. Cook for approximately 5 minutes or until the pears are slightly softened. In a small glass bowl, combine the remaining ¼ cup of water, sugar, and tapioca until they are well mixed. Add the sugar-tapioca mixture to the pears, stirring constantly. Allow to cook for another minute or until the sauce has thickened.

Top each crêpe with ⅛ of the pear mixture and ⅛ of the macadamia cream cheese. Serve immediately.

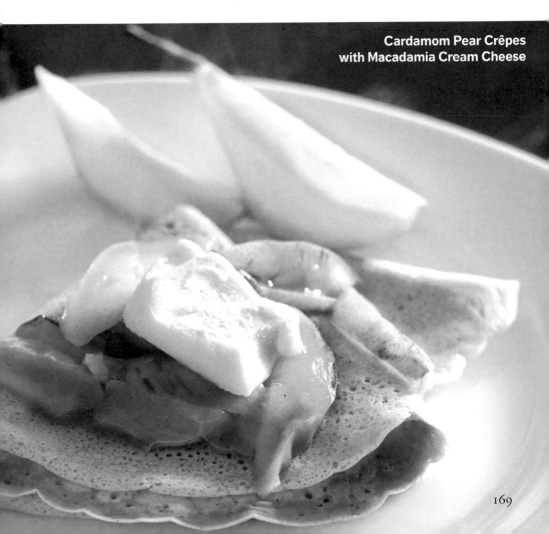

**Cardamom Pear Crêpes
with Macadamia Cream Cheese**

Gingerbread Cookie Ice Cream Sandwiches

The first thing you're probably thinking is "How can fermented gingerbread ice cream sandwiches possibly be good?" Well, they can't be good — they're actually great! The gingerbread cookies are made in a similar way to traditional cookies (and if you eat eggs, you may use 1 large egg in place of the flaxseed-water mixture or Ener-G-water mixture), while the ice cream is made using fermented cashews as the base, which gives it a slight frozen-yogurt taste. These delights quickly took the top spot among my favorite holiday treats! Not only are they absolutely delicious, but they're also gluten-free, dairy-free, and low in sugar (compared to most holiday goodies). After Curtis and I baked up a new batch to fine-tune the recipe, he joked that we'd have to taste-test them too — "in the name of science." And we did. They definitely passed our rigorous scientific testing! Now I am happy to share my new favorite holiday treat with you. But, to be honest, they're so good that I crave them on a hot summer's day as well.

Makes about 24 cookies or 12 ice cream sandwiches with Cultured Vanilla Ice Cream

½ cup coconut oil
½ cup coconut sugar
¼ cup molasses
1 tablespoon finely ground flaxseed whisked into 3 tablespoons water, or 1½ teaspoons
　　Ener-G Egg Replacer whisked into 2 tablespoons water
1 cup brown rice flour
1 cup millet flour
1½ teaspoons baking soda
2 teaspoons ground ginger
1 teaspoon ground cinnamon
¼ teaspoon ground nutmeg
Cultured Vanilla Ice Cream (see page 172)

Preheat your oven to 350°F.

In a mixer, combine the oil and sugar, and begin mixing. While they're still blending, add the molasses, flaxseed-water mixture or Ener-G-water mixture, brown rice flour, millet flour, baking soda, ginger, cinnamon, and nutmeg, and continue to mix until the mixture forms a soft, pliable dough.

Form the dough into balls approximately 1½ inches in diameter, or the size of a walnut. Press them firmly with the palm of your hand onto a parchment-lined baking sheet to form 2-inch disks, leaving space between the cookies for them to spread. Bake for 8 minutes or until they are firm but not hard. Let cool on wire racks.

Once the gingerbread cookies have cooled, spoon the cultured vanilla ice cream onto one of the cookies, and press another cookie onto it to form a sandwich. Repeat for the remaining cookies. Freeze or serve immediately. If freezing, allow the ice cream sandwiches to sit at room temperature for about 10 minutes before serving.

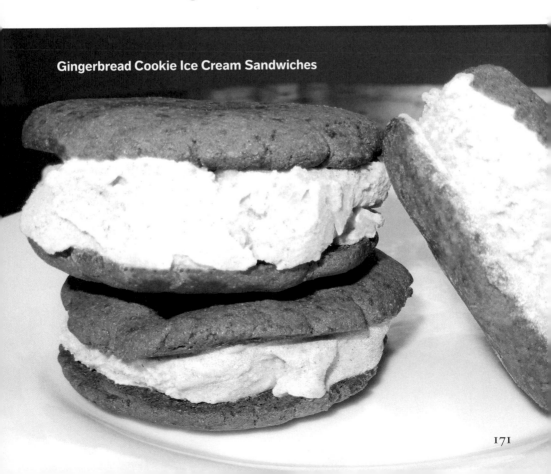

Gingerbread Cookie Ice Cream Sandwiches

Cultured Vanilla Ice Cream

This vanilla ice cream is completely dairy-free but is still delightfully creamy and decadent. You'll enjoy this delicious treat on its own, served with your favorite fruit (it is wonderful with fresh, pitted cherries), or as a sandwich filling for my Gingerbread Cookie Ice Cream Sandwiches (see page 170).

1 cup raw, unsalted cashews
2 cups almond milk (I use unsweetened, but vanilla or sweetened versions are also fine), divided
1 probiotic capsule or ¼ teaspoon probiotic powder
5 large fresh Medjool dates, pitted (if you can't find fresh, use 6 pitted, dried Medjool dates soaked in water for at least a few hours)
1 teaspoon vanilla powder (alternatively, use the seeds scraped from one vanilla bean, or 1 to 2 teaspoons pure vanilla extract)

In a small bowl, combine the cashews and 1 cup of milk; add the contents of the probiotic capsule (discarding the empty capsule shell) or probiotic powder, and mix well. Cover and let sit for eight to twelve hours, depending on your taste preference; longer fermentation times create a tangier flavor.

In a blender, combine the cashew mixture, dates, and vanilla powder, and blend until smooth. Pour into an ice cream machine, and follow the manufacturer's directions to process into ice cream (usually 20 to 25 minutes).

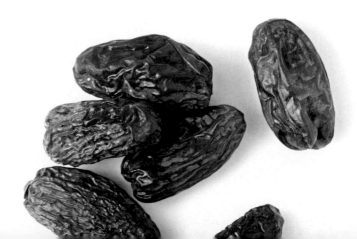

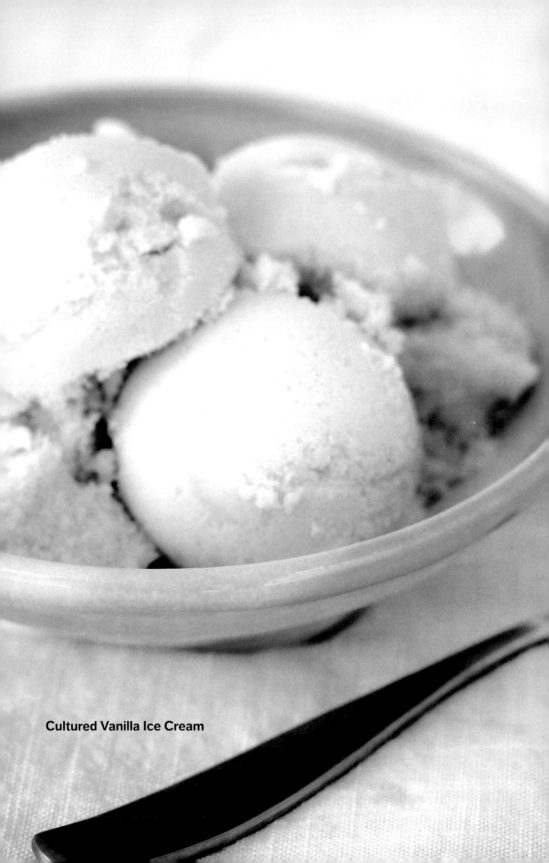

Cultured Vanilla Ice Cream

Pumpkin Pie Ice Cream

Last summer Curtis fenced in our front yard and dug up the grass in preparation for planting a large food garden. Because we live in a natural setting, we needed the fence to keep out deer and deter the bears. When my first planting of squash seeds didn't grow, I planted another batch. Then I decided that growing squash down the retaining wall at the back of our home might also be nice (which it was!). Then, to my surprise, all three batches of squash seeds grew into a wide variety of gorgeous organic squashes. So I began creating new and different ways to enjoy this vegetable. Imagine my anticipation when I created this recipe and then waited for the ice cream maker to churn out the finished product. Then there was the first bite. It was heavenly! I had created my new and favorite way to enjoy squash — in ice cream. Every day after that Curtis and I enjoyed this delightful treat, which doesn't actually contain pumpkins due to my overflow of squash, but tastes like creamy pumpkin pie without the crust, or perhaps even better.

Makes about 1 quart/liter

½ cup raw, unsalted cashews
¼ cup filtered water
2 probiotic capsules, or ½ teaspoon probiotic powder
2 cups almond milk
2 cups cooked squash (such as kabocha, acorn, hubbard, or butternut)
    or 1½ cups pureed cooked squash
7 fresh Medjool dates, pitted
1½ teaspoons ground cinnamon
½ teaspoon ground ginger
½ teaspoon ground cloves
⅛ teaspoon nutmeg

In a small bowl, mix the cashews and water; add the contents of the probiotic capsule (discarding the empty capsule shell) or probiotic powder, and mix well. Cover and let sit for twelve hours.

In a blender, combine the cashew mixture with the milk, squash, dates, cinnamon, ginger. cloves, and nutmeg, and blend until the mixture is smooth. Pour it into an ice cream maker, and follow the manufacturer's instructions. Serve immediately.

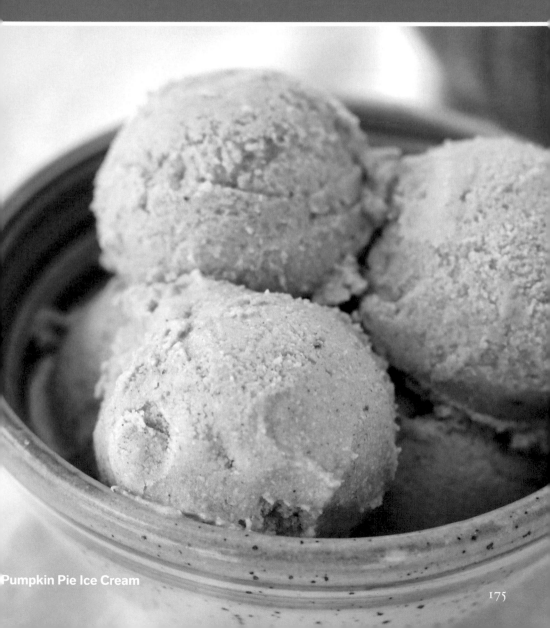

Pumpkin Pie Ice Cream

Black Cherry Ice Cream

By now you may have guessed that I'm a bit of a fermented foods addict. Eating fermented foods makes me feel great, and I love the delicious and unique flavors fermentation creates. After I started experimenting with fermented foods, I soon realized that it would be wonderful to enjoy more fermented desserts. I only indulge in sweets occasionally, but I knew I would feel better about doing so if they offered the health benefits of fermentation. When our friend Larry asked if Curtis and I would like to come by his place to pick cherries from the cherry trees in his yard, I immediately thought of the cultured black cherry ice cream we could eat afterward. You're going to love this delightful recipe.

Makes about 1 quart/liter

1 cup raw, unsalted cashews
1 cup filtered water
1 probiotic capsule or ¼ teaspoon probiotic powder
2 cups fresh black cherries, pitted and stems removed (if using frozen cherries, allow to thaw before using), plus a few more for garnish (optional)
1¼ cup almond milk
4 fresh medjool dates, pitted

In a medium bowl, soak cashews in the water for eight hours or overnight.

Pour the cashews and water into a blender, and blend until the mixture is smooth and creamy. Pour it into a small glass dish with a lid. Empty the probiotic capsule (discarding the empty capsule shell) or probiotic powder into the cashew mixture, and stir together. Cover it with a lid or clean cloth, and allow it to ferment for eight to twelve hours.

In a blender or food processor, combine the cashew mixture with the cherries, milk, and dates, and blend until smooth. Pour the mixture into an ice cream maker, and follow the manufacturer's directions to process into ice cream. Garnish with additional cherries if desired, and serve immediately.

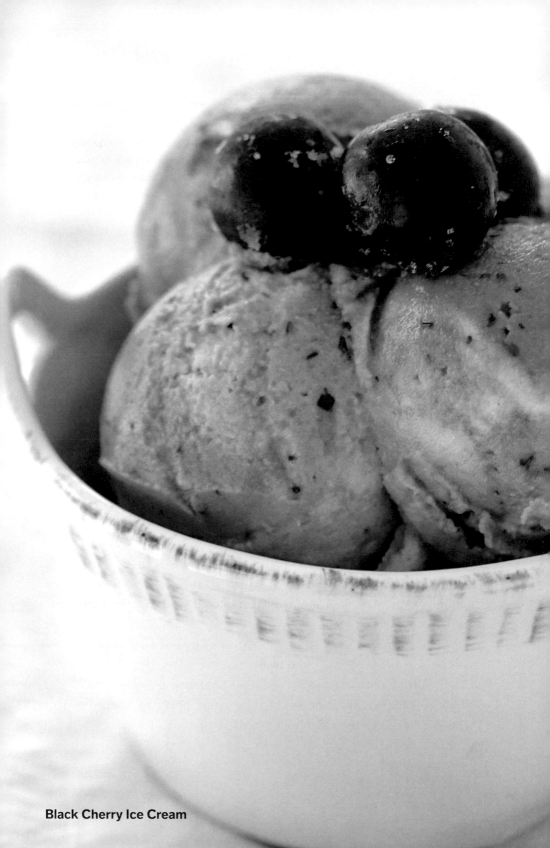

Black Cherry Ice Cream

Orange Creamsicle Cheesecake

This dairy-free, no-bake cheesecake is as good as the real thing. I'm torn between it and the Pomegranate Cheesecake (page 180) as to which one is my favorite. It takes only about thirty minutes to make once all the ingredients are ready, but it does require some inactive time: twelve to twenty-four hours to allow the cashews to ferment, and then four to six hours for the cheesecake to set in the fridge.

Makes one 12-inch cheesecake

Crust

1 cup raw, unsalted almonds
3 fresh Medjool dates, pitted
1 tablespoon coconut oil
Pinch unrefined sea salt

Filling

2 cups raw, unsalted cashews
1 cup filtered water
1 probiotic capsule or ¼ teaspoon probiotic powder
3 cups orange juice
2 tablespoons pure maple syrup
1 teaspoon vanilla powder
1 cup coconut oil
¼ cup plus 1 tablespoon lecithin (5 tablespoons)
Thin slices of orange, with peel, for garnish (optional)

For the crust, in a food processor, combine all crust ingredients, and blend until finely chopped. Transfer to a 12-inch springform pan, and press over the bottom surface of the pan until it is firm.

For the filling, in a medium bowl, combine the cashews, water, and the contents of the probiotic capsule (discarding the empty capsule shell) or probiotic powder; stir until combined. Cover with a lid or clean cloth, and let sit for twelve to twenty-four hours to culture.

In a blender, combine the cashew mixture with the orange juice, maple syrup, vanilla powder, oil, and lecithin, and blend until smooth.

Pour the mixture over the crust. Refrigerate for four to six hours, or until set. Garnish with orange slices if desired, and serve. The cheesecake lasts approximately four days in the refrigerator in a covered container.

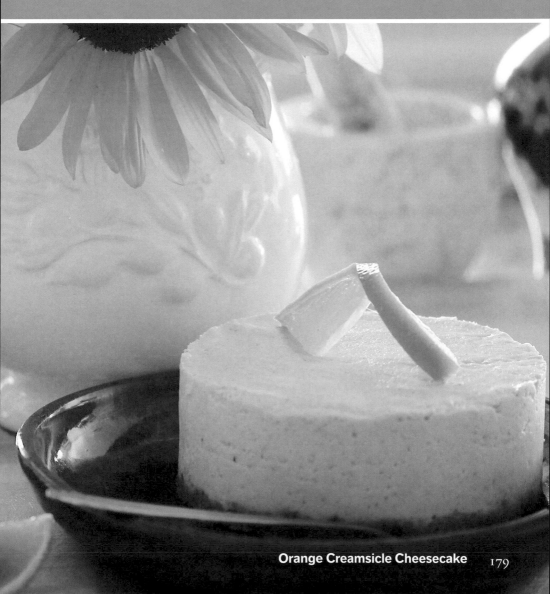

Orange Creamsicle Cheesecake 179

Dairy-Free Pomegranate Cheesecake

This is one of my favorite desserts. It is dairy-free, vegan, and gluten-free, but it contains all the flavor of a traditional cheesecake. Plus, it is packed with the antioxidants naturally found in pomegranates, known as polyphenols. They have anticancerous properties, and help to protect you against heart disease as well as brain disease. This no-bake cheesecake is as good as the real thing. It takes only about thirty minutes to make once all the ingredients are ready, but it does require some inactive time: twelve to twenty-four hours to allow the cashews to ferment and then four to six hours for the cheesecake to set in the fridge.

Makes one 12-inch cheesecake

Crust

1 cup raw, unsalted hazelnuts
4 fresh Medjool dates, pitted
1 tablespoon coconut oil
Pinch unrefined sea salt

Filling

2 cups raw, unsalted cashews
1 cup filtered water
1 probiotic capsule or ¼ teaspoon probiotic powder
3 cups pomegranate juice
2 tablespoons pure maple syrup or agave nectar
1 teaspoon vanilla powder
1 cup coconut oil
¼ cup plus 2 tablespoons lecithin (6 tablespoons)
Fresh pomegranate arils (seeds) to garnish (optional)

For the crust, in a food processor, combine all crust ingredients, and blend until finely chopped. Transfer to a 12-inch springform pan, and press over the bottom surface of the pan until it is firm.

For the filling, in a medium bowl, combine the cashews, water, and the contents of the probiotic capsule (discarding the empty capsule shell) or probiotic powder. Stir the mixture until it is combined. Cover with a lid or clean cloth, and let sit for twelve to twenty-four hours to culture.

In a blender, combine the cashew mixture with the pomegranate juice, maple syrup or agave nectar, vanilla powder, oil, and lecithin, and blend until smooth.

Pour the mixture over the crust. Refrigerate for four to six hours, or until set. Top with fresh pomegranate arils if desired. Serve. The cheesecake lasts approximately four days in the refrigerator in a covered container.

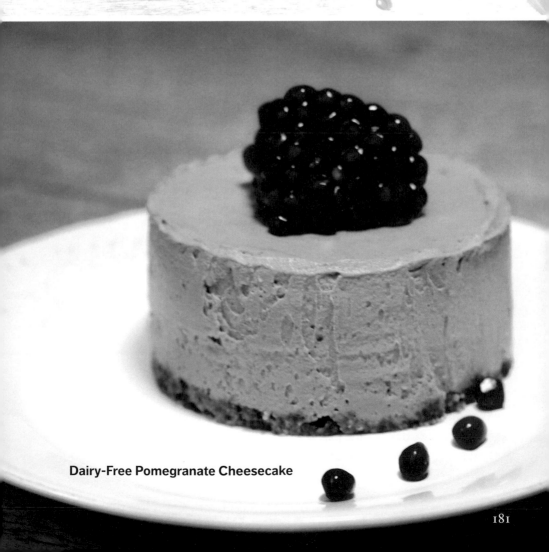

Dairy-Free Pomegranate Cheesecake

Blackberry Cheesecake

This dairy-free, no-bake cheesecake is creamy, delicious, and has the cream cheese–like texture you want in a cheesecake. It takes only about thirty minutes to make once all the ingredients are ready, but it does require some inactive time: one to two days to allow the cashews to ferment and four to six hours for the cheesecake to set in the fridge.

Makes one 12-inch cheesecake

Crust

1 cup raw, unsalted almonds
3 fresh Medjool dates, pitted
1 tablespoon coconut oil
Pinch unrefined sea salt

Filling

2 cups raw, unsalted cashews
1 cup filtered water
1 probiotic capsule or ¼ teaspoon probiotic powder
¼ cup plus 1 tablespoon pure maple syrup (5 tablespoons)
1 teaspoon vanilla powder
½ cup coconut oil
½ cup lecithin
2 cups almond milk
2½ cups fresh blackberries (if using frozen, allow them to thaw before making the cheesecake), plus more for garnish (optional)

For the crust, in a food processor, combine all crust ingredients, and blend until finely chopped. Transfer to a 12-inch springform pan, and press over the bottom surface of the pan until it is firm.

For the filling, in a medium bowl, combine the cashews, water, and the contents of the probiotic capsule (discarding the empty capsule shell) or

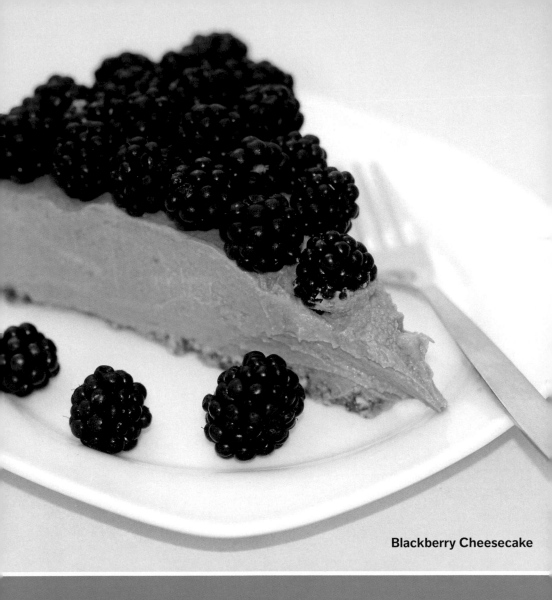

Blackberry Cheesecake

probiotic powder; stir the mixture until it is combined. Cover with a lid or clean cloth, and let sit for twenty-four to forty-eight hours to culture.

In a blender, combine the cashew mixture with the maple syrup, vanilla powder, oil, lecithin, and milk, and blend until smooth. Add the blackberries, and blend until smooth.

Pour the mixture over the crust. Refrigerate for four to six hours, or until set. Garnish with additional blackberries, if desired, and serve. The cheesecake lasts approximately four days in the refrigerator in a covered container.

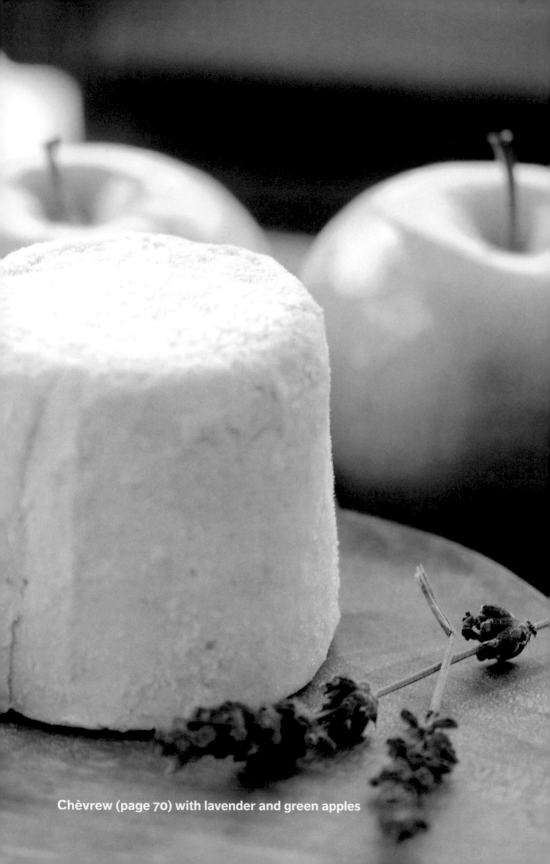

Chèvrew (page 70) with lavender and green apples

ACKNOWLEDGMENTS

Thank you to the many wonderful people involved in making this book happen, specifically:

Georgia Hughes, Munro Magruder, Kristen Cashman, Tristy Taylor, Monique Muhlenkamp, Kim Corbin, Tona Pearce Myers, Tracy Cunningham, Ami Parkerson, and the whole team at New World Library. You're a visionary group and a pleasure to work with.

Josephine Mariea, for your excellent editing work on this project.

Michael and Deborah Schoffro, my wonderful parents, for your ongoing support and belief in me.

Chef Karen McAthy at Blue Heron Creamery for taking the time to be interviewed for this book and sharing your cheese-making secrets.

Alanah Wood, my friend and potter at Woodland Srap Studio, for many of the gorgeous pieces of pottery that grace these pages.

Anita Santos, for coming up with the name "Chèvrew" for my chèvre-like creation (and just for being such a lovely friend).

Curtis Cook, my amazing husband and soulmate, for your immense help in staging the photos, cleaning up the endless food messes afterward, your ongoing support, and for always treating me like a queen and supporting me in all that I do.

NOTES

Chapter 1. Fermented Foods:
The Missing Ingredient to Amazing Health

1. E. Scarpellini, M. Campanale, D. Leone, F. Purchiaroni, G. Vitale, E. C. Lauritano, and A. Gasbarrini, "Gut Microbiota and Obesity," *Internal and Emergency Medicine* 5, suppl. 1 (October 2010): S53–56, www.ncbi.nlm.nih.gov/pubmed/20865475, accessed January 17, 2017.

2. M. Popova, P. Molimard, S. Courau, J. Crociani, C. Dufour, F. Le Vacon, and T. Carton, "Beneficial Effects of Probiotics in Upper Respiratory Tract Infections and Their Mechanical Actions to Antagonize Pathogens," *Journal of Applied Microbiology* 113, no. 6 (December 2012): 1305–18, www.ncbi.nlm.nih.gov/pubmed/22788970, accessed January 17, 2017.

3. M. Tamura, T. Shikina, T. Morihana, M. Hayama, O. Kajimoto, A. Sakamoto, Y. Kajimoto et al., "Effects of Probiotics on Allergic Rhinitis Induced by Japanese Cedar Pollen: Randomized, Double-blind, Placebo-controlled Clinical Trial," *International Archives of Allergy and Immunology* 143, no. 1 (2007): 75–82, www.ncbi.nlm.nih.gov/pubmed/17199093, accessed January 17, 2017.

4. Ibid.

5. US Food and Drug Administration, "Battle of the Bugs: Fighting Antibiotic Resistance," www.fda.gov/Drugs/ResourcesForYou/Consumers/ucm143568.htm, accessed February 3, 2017.

6. E. P. Iakovenko, P. I. Grigor'ev, A. V. Iakovenko, N. A. Agafonova, A. S. Prian-ishnikova, E. N. Sheregova, I. V. Vasil'ev et al., "Effects of Probiotic Bifiform on Efficacy of *Helicobacter pylori* Infection Treatment," *Terapevticheskii Arkhiv* 78, no 2 (2006): 21–26, www.ncbi.nlm.nih.gov/pubmed/16613091, accessed February 3, 2017.

7. G. Reid, D. Charbonneau, J. Erb, B. Kochanowski, D. Beuerman, R. Poehner, and A. W. Bruce, "Oral Use of *Lactobacillus rhamnosus GL-1* and *L. fermentum RC-14* Sig-nificantly Alters Vaginal Flora: Randomized, Placebo-controlled Trial in 64 Healthy Women," *FEMS Immunology and Medical Microbiology* 35, no. 2 (March 20, 2003): 131–34, www.ncbi.nlm.nih.gov/pubmed/12628548, accessed February 3, 2017.

8. Nina Lincoff, "Gut Bacteria May Cause Inflammation in Rheumatoid Arthritis," *Healthline News*, November 8, 2013, www.healthline.com/health-news/arthritis -gut-bacteria-may-trigger-ra-110813, accessed January 17, 2017.

9. J. Liu, J. Sun, F. Wang, X. Yu, Z. Ling, H. Li, H. Zhang et al., "Neuroprotective Effects of *Clostridium butyricum* against Vascular Dementia in Mice via Metabolic Butyrate," *BioMed Research International* (2015): 412946, www.ncbi.nlm.nih.gov /pubmed/26523278, accessed January 17, 2017.

10. M. Perbaglou, J. Katz, R. J. de Souza, J. C. Stearns, M. Motamed, and P. Ritvo, "Pro-biotic Supplementation Can Positively Affect Anxiety and Depressive Symptoms: A Systematic Review of Randomized Controlled Trials," *Nutrition Research* 36, no. 9 (September 2016): 889–98, www.ncbi.nlm.nih.gov/pubmed/27632908, ac-cessed February 3, 2017.

11. X. Hu, T. Wang, and F. Jin, "Alzheimer's Disease and Gut Microbiota," *Science China. Life Sciences* 59, no. 10 (October 2016): 1006–23, www.ncbi.nlm.nih.gov /pubmed/27566465, accessed February 3, 2017.

12. Matthew Hilimire, Jordan E. DeVylder, and Catherine A. Forestell, "Fermented Foods, Neuroticism, and Social Anxiety: An Interactive Model," *Psychiatry Re-search* 228, no. 2 (August 15, 2015): 203–8, www.psy-journal.com/article/S0165-1781%2815%2900214-0/abstract, accessed February 3, 2017.

13. Traci Pedersen, "Fermented Foods Linked to Decreased Social Anxiety," *PsychCen-tral*, June 12, 2015, https://psychcentral.com/news/2015/06/12/fermented-foods -linked-to-decreased-social-anxiety/85640.html, accessed February 3, 2017.

14. P. Bercik, E. F. Verdu, J. A. Foster, J. Macri, M. Potter, X. Huang, P. Malinowski et al., "Chronic Gastrointestinal Inflammation Induces Anxiety-like Behavior and Alters Central Nervous System Biochemistry in Mice," *Gastroenterology* 139, no. 6 (December 2010): 2102–12, www.ncbi.nlm.nih.gov/pubmed/20600016, accessed February 3, 2017.

15. M. Messaoudi, R. Lalonde, N. Violle, H. Javelot, D. Desor, A. Nejdi, J. F. Bisson et al., "Assessment of Psychotropic-like Properties of a Probiotic Formulation (*Lac-tobacillus helveticus R0052* and *Bifidobacterium longum R0175*) in Rats and Human Subjects," *British Journal of Nutrition* 105, no. 5 (March 2011): 755–64, www.ncbi.nlm .nih.gov/pubmed/20974015, accessed February 3, 2017.

16. A. Lyra, S. Lahtinen, K. Tiihonen, and A. Ouwehand, "Intestinal Microbiota and Overweight," *Beneficial Microbes* 1, no. 4 (December 14, 2010): 407–21, http://www.wageningenacademic.com/doi/10.3920/BM2010.0030, accessed March 31, 2017.

17. Ibid.

18. Scarpellini et al., "Gut Microbiota and Obesity."

19. Ibid.

20. R. Q. Yu, J. L. Yuan, L. Y. Ma, Q. X. Qin, and X. Y Wu, "Probiotics Improve Obesity-Associated Dyslipidemia and Insulin Resistance in High-fat Diet-fed Rats," *Chinese Journal of Contemporary Pediatrics* 15, no. 12 (December 2013): 1123–27, www.ncbi.nlm.nih.gov/pubmed/24342213, accessed March 31, 2017.

21. M. S. Kaya, F. Bayiroglu, L. Mis, D. Kilinc, and B. Comba, "In Case of Obesity, Longevity-related Mechanisms Lead to Anti-inflammation," *Age* 36, no. 2 (April 2014): 677–87, www.ncbi.nlm.nih.gov/pubmed/24306820, accessed March 31, 2017.

22. J. E. Park, S. H. Oh, and Y. S. Cha. "*Lactobacillus plantarum LG42* Isolated from Gajami Sik-hae Decreases Body and Fat Pad Weights in Diet-induced Obese Mice," *Journal of Applied Microbiology* 116, no. 1 (January 2014): 145–56, www.ncbi.nlm.nih.gov/pubmed/24131682, accessed March 31, 2017.

23. L. V. Mosiichuk, "Assessment of Safety and Effectiveness of Dietary Fermented Milk Product Using in the Presence of Dysbiosis in People with Overweight and Obesity," *Voprosy Pitaniia* 82, no. 2 (2013): 37–41, www.ncbi.nlm.nih.gov/pubmed/24000698, accessed March 31, 2017.

24. Yu et al., "Probiotics Improve Obesity-associated Dyslipidemia and Insulin Resistance in High-fat Diet-fed Rats."

25. K. K. Sharafedtinov, O. A. Plotnikova, R. I. Alexeeva, T. B. Sentsova, E. Songisepp, J. Stsepetova, I. Smidt et al., "Hypocaloric Diet Supplemented with Probiotic Cheese Improves Body Mass Index and Blood Pressure Indices of Obese Hypertensive Patients: A Randomized Double-blind Placebo-controlled Pilot Study," *Nutrition Journal* 12 (October 12, 2013): 138, www.ncbi.nlm.nih.gov/pubmed/24120179, accessed March 31, 2017.

26. M. Miyoshi, A Ogawa, S. Higurashi, and Y. Kadooka, "Anti-obesity Effect of *Lactobacillus gasseri SBT2055* Accompanied by Inhibition of Pro-inflammatory Gene Expression in the Visceral Adipose Tissue in Diet-induced Obese Mice," *European Journal of Nutrition* 53, no. 2 (2014): 599–606, www.ncbi.nlm.nih.gov/pubmed/23917447, accessed March 31, 2017.

27. M. C. Mekkes, T. C. Weenen, R. J. Brummer, and E. Claassen, "The Development of Probiotic Treatment in Obesity: A Review," *Beneficial Microbes* 5, no 1 (March 2014): 19–28, www.ncbi.nlm.nih.gov/pubmed/23886977, accessed March 31, 2017.

28. Alison Evert, "Phytochemicals," *MedlinePlus*, May 5, 2011, www.nlm.nih.gov/medlineplus/ency/imagepages/19303.htm, accessed March 31, 2017.

29. Kun-Young Park, Ji-Kang Jeong, Yong-Eun Lee, and James W. Daily, "Health

Benefits of Kimchi (Korean Fermented Vegetables) as a Probiotic Food," *Journal of Medicinal Food* 17, no 1 (January 2014): 6–20, www.ncbi.nlm.nih.gov/pubmed /24456350, accessed March 31, 2017.

30. A. Ito, H. Watanabe, and N. Basaran, "Effects of Soy Products in Reducing Risk of Spontaneous and Neutron-Induced Liver Tumors in Mice," *International Journal of Oncology* 2, no. 5 (May 1993): 773–76, www.spandidos-publications.com /ijo/2/5/773, accessed March 31, 2017; K. Shiraki, K. Une, R. Yano, S. Otani, A. Mimeoka, and H. Watanabe, "Inhibition by Long-Term Fermented Miso of Induction of Pulmonary Adenocarcinoma by Diisopropanolnitrosamine in Wistar Rats," *Hiroshima Journal of Medical Science* 52, no. 1 (March 2003): 9–13, www.ncbi.nlm.nih .gov/pubmed/12701648, accessed March 31, 2017.

31. F. M. Barreto, A. N. Colado Simão, H. K. Morimoto, M. A. Batisti Lozovoy, I. Dichi, and H. Da Silva Miglioranza, "Beneficial Effects of *Lactobacillus plantarum* on Glycemia and Homocysteine Levels in Postmenopausal Women with Metabolic Syndrome," *Nutrition* 30, no. 7–8 (July–August 2014): 939–42, www.ncbi.nlm.nih.gov /pubmed/24613434, accessed March 31, 2017.

32. Eva M. Selhub, Alan C. Logan, and Alison C. Bested, "Fermented Foods, Microbiota, and Mental Health: Ancient Practice Meets Nutritional Psychiatry," *Journal of Physiological Anthropology* 33, no. 1 (January 15, 2014): 2, www.ncbi.nlm.nih.gov /pmc/articles/PMC3904694, accessed March 31, 2017.

33. Shiraki et al., "Inhibition by Long-Term Fermented Miso of Induction of Pulmonary Adenocarcinoma by Diisopropanolnitrosamine in Wistar Rats."

34. Lyra et al., "Intestinal Microbiota and Overweight."

35. NIH Human Microbiome Project, http://hmpdacc.org, accessed November 28, 2016.

36. X. W. Gao, M. Mubasher, C. Y. Fang, C. Reifer, and L. E. Miller, "Dose-response Efficacy of a Proprietary Probiotic Formula of *Lactobacillus acidophilus CL1285* and *Lactobacillus casei LBC80-R* for Antibiotic-associated Diarrhea and Clostridium difficile-associated Diarrhea Prophylaxis in Adult Patients," *American Journal of Gastroenterology* 105, no. 7 (July 2010): 1636–41, www.ncbi.nlm.nih.govpubmed /20145608, accessed February 3, 2017; E. Lonnermark, V. Friman, G. Lappas, T. Sandbert, A. Berggren, and I. Adlerberth, "Intake of *Lactobacillus plantarum* Reduces Certain Gastrointestinal Symptoms During Treatment with Antibiotics," *Journal of Clinical Gastroenterology* 44, no. 2 (February 2010): 106–12, www.ncbi.nlm.nih.gov /pubmed/19727002, accessed March 31, 2017.

37. A. Lyra, S. Forssten, P. Rolny, Y. Wettergren, S. J. Lahtinen, K. Salli, L. Cedgård et al., "Comparison of Bacterial Quantities in Left and Right Colon Biopsies and Faeces," *World Journal of Gastroenterology* 18, no. 32 (August 28, 2012): 4404–11, www.ncbi.nlm.nih.gov/pubmed/22969206, accessed February 3, 2017.

Chapter 2. Dairy-Free Yogurt

1. "Yogurt," Wikipedia, https://en.wikipedia.org/wiki/Yogurt.

2. Barreto et al., "Beneficial Effects of *Lactobacillus plantarum* on Glycemia and Homocysteine Levels in Postmenopausal Women with Metabolic Syndrome."

3. E. Guillemard, F. Tondu, F. Lacoin, and J. Schrezenmeir, "Consumption of a Fermented Dairy Product Containing the Probiotic *Lactobacillus casei DN-114001* Reduces the Duration of Respiratory Infections in the Elderly in a Randomised Controlled Trial," *British Journal of Nutrition* 103, no. 1 (January 2010): 58–68, www.ncbi .nlm.nih.gov/pubmed/19747410, accessed March 31, 2017; K. Ohsawa, N. Uchida, K. Ohki, Y. Nakamura, and H. Yokogoshi, "*Lactobacillus helveticus*-fermented Milk Improves Learning and Memory in Mice," *Nutritional Neuroscience* 18, no. 5 (July 2015): 232–40, www.ncbi.nlm.nih.gov/pubmed/24694020, accessed March 31, 2017; F. Aragon et al., "The Administration of Milk Fermented by the Probiotic *Lactobacillus casei CRL 431* Exerts an Immunomodulatory Effect against a Breast Tumour in a Mouse Model," *Immunobiology* 219, no. 6 (June 2014): 457–64, www.ncbi.nlm.nih .gov/pubmed/24646876, accessed March 31, 2017.

4. Guillemard et al., "Consumption of a Fermented Dairy Product Containing the Probiotic *Lactobacillus casei DN-114001* Reduces the Duration of Respiratory Infections in the Elderly in a Randomised Controlled Trial."

5. E. Guillemard, J. Tanguy, A. Flavigny, S. de la Motte, and J. Schrezenmeir, "Effects of Consumption of a Fermented Dairy Product Containing the Probiotic *Lactobacillus casei DN-114001* on Common Respiratory and Gastrointestinal Infections in Shift Workers in a Randomized Controlled Trial," *Journal of the American College of Nutrition* 29, no. 5 (October 2010): 455–68, www.ncbi.nlm.nih.gov/pubmed/21504972, accessed March 31, 2017.

6. P. Timan, N. Rojanasthien, M. Manorot, C. Sangdee, and S. Teekachunhatean, "Effect of Symbiotic Fermented Milk on Oral Bioavailabilty of Isoflavones in Postmenopausal Women," *International Journal of Food Science and Nutrition* 65, no. 6 (September 2014): 761–67, www.ncbi.nlm.nih.gov/pubmed/24720601, accessed March 31, 2017.

7. Aragon et al., "The Administration of Milk Fermented by the Probiotic *Lactobacillus casei CRL 431* Exerts an Immunomodulatory Effect against a Breast Tumour in a Mouse Model."

8. A. Sachdeva, S. Rawat, and J. Nagpal, "Efficacy of Fermented Milk and Whey Proteins in *Helicobacter pylori* Eradication: A Review," *World Journal of Gastroenterology* 20, no. 3 (January 21, 2014): 724–37, www.ncbi.nlm.nih.gov/pubmed/24574746, accessed March 31, 2017.

9. E. Zagato, E. Mileti, L. Massimiliano, F. Fasano, A. Budelli, G. Penna, and M. Rescigno, "*Lactobacillus paracasei CBA L74* Metabolic Products and Fermented

Milk for Infant Formula Have Anti-inflammatory Activity on Dendritic Cells in Vitro and Protective Effects against Colitis and an Enteric Pathogen in Vivo," *PLoS One* 9, no. 2 (February 10, 2014): e87615, www.ncbi.nlm.nih.gov/pubmed/24520333, accessed March 31, 2017.

10. Kazuhito Ohsawa, Naoto Uchida, Kohji Ohki, Yasunori Nakamura, and Hidehiko Yokkogoshi, "*Lactobacillus helveticus*-fermented Milk Improves Learning and Memory in Mice," *Nutritional Neuroscience* 18, no. 5 (July 2015): 232–40, www.ncbi.nlm.nih.gov/pubmed/24694020, accessed March 31, 2017.

11. IuA Siniavskĭ, V. A. Kraĭsman, and ZhM Suleĭmenova, "Using of a Specialized Fermented Soy Milk Product on the Basis of Soybeans in Cardiology Practice," *Viprosy pitaniia* 82, no. 5 (2013): 51–57, www.ncbi.nlm.nih.gov/pubmed/24640160, accessed March 31, 2017; L. R. Lai, S. C. Hsieh, H. Y. Huang, and C. C. Chou, "Effect of Lactic Acid Fermentation on the Total Phenolic, Saponin, and Phytic Acid Contents, as well as Anti-colon Cancer Cell Proliferation Activity of Soy Milk," *Journal of Bioscience and Bioengineering* 115, no. 5 (May 2013): 552–56, www.ncbi.nlm.nih.gov/pubmed/23290992, accessed March 31, 2017.

Chapter 3. Vegan Cheeses

1. S. Bhattacharyya, L. Feferman, T. Unterman, and J. K. Tobacman, "Exposure to Common Food Additive Carrageenan Alone Leads to Fasting Hyperglycemia and in Combination with a High Fat Diet Exacerbates Glucose Intolerance and Hyperlipidemia without Effect on Weight," *Journal of Diabetes Research* (2015): 513429, www.ncbi.nlm.nih.gov/pubmed/25883986, accessed March 31, 2017.

2. Catherine St. Louis, "Warning Too Late for Some Babies," *New York Times*, February 4, 2013, http://well.blogs.nytimes.com/2013/02/04/warning-too-late-for-some-babies/?_r=1.

3. "Update: June 5, 2011: FDA Continues to Investigate Necrotizing Enterocolitis and SimplyThick Following Company's Recall," US Food and Drug Administration, www.fda.gov/NewsEvents/newsroom/PressAnnouncements/ucm256253.htm.

4. J. Beal, B. Silverman, J. Bellant, T. E. Young, and K. Klontz, "Late Onset Necrotizing Enterocolitis in Infants Following Use of a Xanthan Gum-containing Thickening Agent," *Journal of Pediatrics* 161, no. 2 (August 2012): 354–56, www.ncbi.nlm.nih.gov/pubmed?term=beal%20late%20onset%20necrotizing, accessed March 31, 2017.

5. D. L. Trout, R. O. Ryan, and M. C. Bickard, "The Amount and Distribution of Water, Dry Matter and Sugars in the Digestive Tracts of Rats Fed Xanthan Gum," *Proceedings of the Society for Experimental Biology and Medicine* 172, no. 3 (March 1983): 340–45, www.ncbi.nlm.nih.gov/pubmed/6844340, accessed March 31, 2017.

6. J. Daly, J. Tomlin, and N. W. Read, "The Effect of Feeding Xanthan Gum on Colonic Function in Man: Correlation with in Vitro Determinants of Bacterial Breakdown,"

British Journal of Nutrition 69, no. 3 (May 1993): 897–902, www.ncbi.nlm.nih.gov /pubmed/8329363, accessed March 31, 2017.

Chapter 4. Sauerkraut, Pickles, and Cultured Vegetables

1. V. K. Baipai, K. C. Kang, and K. H. Baek, "Microbial Fermentation of Cabbage by a Bacterial Strain of *Pectobacterium atrosepticum* for the Production of Bioactive Material against Candida Species," *Journal de Mycologie Medicale* 22, no. 1 (March 2012): 21–29, www.ncbi.nlm.nih.gov/pubmed/23177810, accessed March 31, 2017.

2. A. W. Nichols, "Probiotics and Athletics: A Systematic Review," *Current Sports Medicine Reports* 6, no. 4 (July 2007): 269–73, www.ncbi.nlm.nih.gov/pubmed/17618005, accessed March 31, 2017.

3. D. Gao, X. Gao, and G. Zhu, "Antioxidant Effects of *Lactobacillus plantarum* via Activation of Transcription Factor Nrf2," *Food and Function* 4, no 6 (June 2013): 982–89, www.ncbi.nlm.nih.gov/pubmed/23681127, accessed March 31, 2017.

4. Y. H. Ju, K. E. Carlson, J. Sun, D. Pathak, B. S. Katzenellenbogen, J. A. Katzenellenbogen, and W. G. Helferich., "Estrogenic Effects of Extracts from Cabbage, Fermented Cabbage, and Acidified Brussels Sprouts, on Growth and Gene Expression of Estrogen-Dependent Human Breast Cancer (MCF) Cells," *Journal of Agriculture and Food Chemistry* 48, no. 10 (October 2000): 4628–34, www.ncbi.nlm.nih.gov/pubmed /11052710, accessed March 31, 2017.

5. J. Cho, D. Lee, C. Yang, J. Jeon, J. Kim and H. Han, "Microbial Population Dynamics of Kimchi, a Fermented Cabbage Product," *FEMS Microbiology Letters* 257, no. 2 (April 2006): 262–67, www.ncbi.nlm.nih.gov/pubmed/16553862, accessed February 3, 2017.

6. J. Kaushik, A. Kumar, R. K. Duary, A. K. Mohanty, S. Grover and V. K. Batish, "Functional and Probiotic Attributes of an Indigenous Isolate of *Lactobacillus plantarum*," *PLoS One* 4, no. 12 (December 1, 2009): e8099, www.ncbi.nlm.nih.gov /pubmed/19956615, accessed February 3, 2017.

7. I. H. Jung, M. A. Jung, E. J. Kim, M. J. Han, and D. H. Kim, "*Lactobacillus pentosus var. plantarum C29* Protects Scopolamine-induced Memory Deficit in Mice," *Journal of Applied Microbiology* 113, no. 6 (December 2012): 1498–506, www.ncbi.nlm.nih.gov /pubmed/22925033, accessed February 3, 2017.

8. Park et al., "Health Benefits of Kimchi (Korean Fermented Vegetables) as a Probiotic Food."

Chapter 5. Fruit Cultures and Homemade Vinegars

1. C. S. Johnston, I. Steplewska, C. A. Long, L. N. Harris, and R. H. Ryals, "Examination of the Antiglycemic Properties of Vinegar in Healthy Adults," *Annals of Nutrition*

and Metabolism 56, no. 1 (2010): 74–79, www.ncbi.nlm.nih.gov/pubmed/20068289, accessed January 20, 2017.

2. F. Shishehbor, A. Mansoori, A. R. Sarkaki, M. T. Jalali, and S. M. Latifi, "Apple Cider Vinegar Attenuates Lipid Profile in Normal and Diabetic Rats," *Pakistani Journal of Biological Sciences* 11, no. 23 (December 1, 2008): 2634–38, www.ncbi.nlm.nih.gov /pubmed/19630216, accessed January 20, 2017.

3. C. Vijayakumar and C. E. Wolf-Hall, "Evaluation of Household Sanitizers for Reducing Levels of *Escherichia coli* on Iceberg Lettuce," *Journal of Food Protection* 65, no. 10 (October 2002): 1646–50, www.ncbi.nlm.nih.gov/pubmed/12380754, accessed January 20, 2017.

4. M. Naziroğlu, M. Güler, C. Özgül, G. Saydam, M. Küçükayaz, and E. Sözbir, "Apple Cider Vinegar Modulates Serum Lipid Profile, Erythrocyte, Kidney and Liver Membrane Oxidative Stress in Ovariectomized Mice Fed High Cholesterol," *Journal of Membrane Biology* 247, no. 8 (August 2014): 667–73, www.ncbi.nlm.nih.gov/pubmed /24894721, accessed January 20, 2017.

5. E. Ostman, Y. Granfeldt, L. Persson, and I. Björck, "Vinegar Supplementation Lowers Glucose and Insulin Responses and Increases Satiety after a Bread Meal in Healthy Subjects," *European Journal of Clinical Nutrition* 59, no. 9 (September 2005): 983–88, www.ncbi.nlm.nih.gov/pubmed/16015276, accessed January 20, 2017.

6. T. Kondo, M. Kishi, T. Fushimi, S. Ugajin, and T. Kaga, "Vinegar Intake Reduces Body Weight, Body Fat Mass, and Serum Triglyceride Levels in Obese Japanese Subjects," *Bioscience, Biotechnology, and Biochemistry* 73, no. 8 (August 2009): 1837–43, www.ncbi.nlm.nih.gov/pubmed/19661687, accessed January 20, 2017.

7. J. A. Laranjinha, L. M. Almeida, and V. M. Madeira, "Reactivity of Dietary Phenolic Acids with Peroxyl Radicals: Antioxidant Activity upon Low Density Lipoprotein Peroxidation," *Biochemical Pharmacology* 48, no. 3 (August 1994): 487–94, www.ncbi .nlm.nih.gov/pubmed/8068036, accessed January 20, 2017.

8. R. Darnelles-Morgental, J. M. Guerreiro-Tanomaru, N. B. de Faria-Júnior, M. A. Hungaro-Duarte, M. C. Kuga, and M. Tanomaru-Filho, "Antibacterial Efficacy of Endodontic Irrigating Solutions and Their Combinations in Root Canals Contaminated by *Enterococcus faecalis*," *Oral Surgery, Oral Medicine, Oral Pathology, Oral Radiology and Endodontics* 112, no. 3 (September 2011): 396–400, www.ncbi.nlm.nih .gov/pubmed/21531598, accessed January 20, 2017.

9. K. Nanda, N. Miyoshi, Y. Nakamura, Y. Shimoji, Y. Tamura, Y. Nishikawa, K. Uenakai et al., "Extract of Vinegar 'Kurosu' from Unpolished Rice Inhibits the Proliferation of Human Cancer Cells," *Journal of Experimental and Clinical Cancer Research* 23, no. 1 (March 2004): 69–75, www.ncbi.nlm.nih.gov/pubmed/15149153, accessed March 31, 2017; A. Mimura, Y. Suzuki, Y. Toshima, S. Yazaki, T. Ohtsuki, S. Ui, and F. Hyodoh, "Induction of Apoptosis in Human Leukemia Cells by Naturally Fermented Sugar Cane Vinegar (Kibizu) of Amami Ohshima Island," *Biofactors*

22, no. 1–4 (2004): 93–97, www.ncbi.nlm.nih.gov/pubmed/15630260, accessed January 20, 2017.

Chapter 6. Cultured Beverages: Vegan Kefir, Kombucha, and More

1. H. Maeda, X. Zhu, K. Omura, S. Suzuki, and S. Kitamura, "Effects of an Exopolysaccharide (Kefiran) on Lipids, Blood Pressure, Blood Glucose, and Constipation," *Biofactors* 22, no. 1–4 (2004): 197–200, www.ncbi.nlm.nih.gov/pubmed/15630283, accessed January 20, 2017.

2. Ibid.

3. Ibid.

4. M. Ghoneum and J. Gimzewski, "Apoptotic Effect of a Novel Kefir Product, PFT, on Multidrug-Resistant Myeloid Leukemia Cells via a Hole-Piercing Mechanism," *International Journal of Oncology* 44, no. 3 (March 2014): 830–37, www.ncbi.nlm.nih.gov/pubmed/24430613, accessed March 31, 2017.

5. I. Vina, P. Semjonovs, R. Linde, and I. Denina, "Current Evidence on Physiological Activity and Expected Health Effects of Kombucha Fermented Beverage," *Journal of Medicinal Food* 17, no. 2 (February 2014): 179–88, www.ncbi.nlm.nih.gov/pubmed/24192111, accessed March 31, 2017.

6. S. Bhattacharya, R. Gachhui, and P. C. Sil, "Effect of Kombucha, a Fermented Black Tea in Attenuating Oxidative Stress Mediated Tissue Damage in Alloxan Induced Diabetic Rats," *Food and Chemical Toxicology* 60 (October 2013): 328–40, www.ncbi.nlm.nih.gov/pubmed/23907022, accessed March 31, 2017.

7. A. J. Marsh, O. O'Sullivan, C. Hill, R. P. Ross, and P. D. Cotter, "Sequence-based Analysis of the Bacterial and Fungal Compositions of Multiple Kombucha (Tea Fungus) Samples," *Food Microbiology* 38 (April 2014): 171–78, www.ncbi.nlm.nih.gov/pubmed/24290641, accessed March 31, 2017.

8. Y. Wang, B. Ji, W. Wu, R. Wang, Z. Yang, D. Zhang, and W. Tian, "Hepatoprotective Effects of Kombucha Tea: Identification of Functional Strains and Quantification of Functional Components," *Journal of the Science of Food and Agriculture* 94, no. 2 (January 30, 2014): 265–72, www.ncbi.nlm.nih.gov/pubmed/23716136, accessed March 31, 2017.

9. D. Bhattacharya, S. Bhattacharya, M. M. Patra, S. Chakravorty, S. Sarkar, W. Chakraborty, H. Koley et al., "Antibacterial Activity of Polyphenolic Fraction of Kombucha against Enteric Bacterial Pathogens," *Current Microbiology* 73, no. 6 (December 2016): 885–96, www.ncbi.nlm.nih.gov/pubmed/27638313, accessed January 27, 2017.

INDEX

ABOUT THE AUTHOR

Michelle Schoffro Cook, PhD, DNM, DHS, ROHP, is the author
of twenty books, including the international bestsellers *60 Seconds to Slim*,
The Ultimate pH Solution, and *The 4-Week Ultimate Body Detox Plan*. Her
books have been translated into many languages, including Spanish, Greek,
Chinese, Thai, Indonesian, and Russian.

Her culinary creations and work have appeared in *Woman's World*, *First
for Women*, *WebMD*, *Huffington Post*, *Mother Earth Living*, *Mother Earth
News*, *Prevention*, *Women's Health*, and *Vegetarian Times*. She is a blogger
for Care2.com, RodaleWellness.com, DrMichelleCook.com, and Cultured-
Cook.com. Dr. Cook has received a World-Leading Intellectual Award for
her contribution to natural medicine.

World's Healthiest News

You can subscribe to Dr. Cook's free e-zine, *World's Healthiest News*, to obtain natural health insights, news, research, recipes, and more. Each edition
features natural approaches to boost your energy, supercharge your immune
system, and look and feel great. Subscribe at WorldsHealthiestDiet.com or
DrMichelleCook.com.

Dr. Cook's Blogs

Don't miss a single blog post by Dr. Cook. Follow her at:

DrMichelleCook.com
CulturedCook.com
Care2.com/GreenLiving/author/MCook
Facebook.com/DrSchoffroCook
Twitter @mschoffrocook
Pinterest.com/DrMichelleCook
Instagram.com/DrMichelleCook

Discover Dr. Cook's exclusive ebooks at:

WorldsHealthiestDiet.com

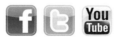
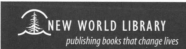